Drugs and Sports

Peggy J. Parks

Current Issues

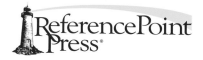
ReferencePoint
Press®

San Diego, CA

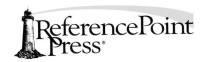

© 2010 ReferencePoint Press, Inc.

For more information, contact:
ReferencePoint Press, Inc.
PO Box 27779
San Diego, CA 92198
www.ReferencePointPress.com

Picture credits:
Cover: Dreamstime and iStockphoto.com
Maury Aaseng: 31-34, 46–48, 60–63, 76–78
AP Images: 10, 15

LIBRARY OF CONGRESS CATALOGING-IN-PUBLICATION DATA

Parks, Peggy J., 1951–
    Drugs and sports / by Peggy J. Parks.
        p. cm. — (Compact research series)
    Includes bibliographical references and index.
    ISBN-13: 978-1-60152-105-7 (hardback)
    ISBN-10: 1-60152-105-7 (hardback)
    1. Doping in sports. 2. Athletes—Drug use. 3. Drug testing. I. Title.
    RC1230.P37   2009
    362.29—dc22
                                                        2009036847-

Contents

Foreword

66Where is the knowledge we have lost in information?99

—T.S. Eliot, "The Rock."

As modern civilization continues to evolve, its ability to create, store, distribute, and access information expands exponentially. The explosion of information from all media continues to increase at a phenomenal rate. By 2020 some experts predict the worldwide information base will double every 73 days. While access to diverse sources of information and perspectives is paramount to any democratic society, information alone cannot help people gain knowledge and understanding. Information must be organized and presented clearly and succinctly in order to be understood. The challenge in the digital age becomes not the creation of information, but how best to sort, organize, enhance, and present information.

ReferencePoint Press developed the *Compact Research* series with this challenge of the information age in mind. More than any other subject area today, researching current issues can yield vast, diverse, and unqualified information that can be intimidating and overwhelming for even the most advanced and motivated researcher. The *Compact Research* series offers a compact, relevant, intelligent, and conveniently organized collection of information covering a variety of current topics ranging from illegal immigration and deforestation to diseases such as anorexia and meningitis.

The series focuses on three types of information: objective single-author narratives, opinion-based primary source quotations, and facts and statistics. The clearly written objective narratives provide context and reliable background information. Primary source quotes are carefully selected and cited, exposing the reader to differing points of view. And facts and statistics sections aid the reader in evaluating perspectives. Presenting these key types of information creates a richer, more balanced learning experience.

For better understanding and convenience, the series enhances information by organizing it into narrower topics and adding design features that make it easy for a reader to identify desired content. For example, in *Compact Research: Illegal Immigration*, a chapter covering the economic impact of illegal immigration has an objective narrative explaining the various ways the economy is impacted, a balanced section of numerous primary source quotes on the topic, followed by facts and full-color illustrations to encourage evaluation of contrasting perspectives.

The ancient Roman philosopher Lucius Annaeus Seneca wrote, "It is quality rather than quantity that matters." More than just a collection of content, the *Compact Research* series is simply committed to creating, finding, organizing, and presenting the most relevant and appropriate amount of information on a current topic in a user-friendly style that invites, intrigues, and fosters understanding.

Drugs and Sports at a Glance

Drugs Used by Athletes

The most common drugs used by athletes are those that enhance sports performance, such as steroids and human growth hormone. Some athletes have also tested positive for drugs such as marijuana, cocaine, and methamphetamine, which are illegal under federal law.

Performance-Enhancing Drugs and the Law

In the United States steroids and human growth hormone may be prescribed by physicians but only to treat medical conditions. People who take the drugs for nonmedical conditions (such as to enhance sports performance) are doing so illegally.

What Steroids Do

Steroids, which may be injected or taken orally, boost athletic performance by causing muscles to grow faster and by increasing muscle mass and strength.

Health Risks

A number of serious risks have been associated with performance-enhancing drugs. Side effects include liver and kidney damage, heart disease, and high blood pressure, as well as severe acne on the body.

Seriousness of Problem

Drug use occurs in numerous sports and at all levels, from student athletes to Olympic and professional athletes. The exact number of athletes who use drugs cannot be determined because there is no way to know how many escape being caught.

Drug Testing for Students

Only New Jersey, Texas, and Illinois have statewide drug-testing policies for student athletes, although many schools in other states have implemented their own policies. College drug policies are overseen by the National Collegiate Athletic Association.

Drug Testing for Olympic and Professional Athletes

The World Anti-Doping Agency has tough drug policies in place for Olympic athletes, and violators face stiff punishments if they are caught using drugs. Professional sports organizations often have tough policies, too, but they are free to make their own decisions about drug testing.

Legalization Issue

Those who want performance-enhancing drugs to remain illegal say that people who take the drugs have an unfair advantage and are cheating. Those who advocate for legalizing the drugs say they are just another means of increasing competitiveness and that adult athletes should be able to decide for themselves whether or not to use them.

Overview

❝For more than a decade there has been widespread illegal use of anabolic steroids and other performance enhancing substances by players in Major League Baseball, in violation of federal law and baseball policy.❞

—George J. Mitchell, a former U.S. senator from Maine who investigated the use of performance-enhancing drugs among professional baseball players.

❝I don't need the Hall of Fame to justify that I put my butt on the line and I worked my tail off. And I defy anybody to say I did it by cheating or taking any shortcuts.❞

—Roger Clemens, a Major League Baseball pitcher who was named in a December 2007 congressional report as one of the athletes who had used performance-enhancing drugs.

In October 2007, 5-time Olympic medalist Marion Jones made a confession that shocked sports fans everywhere. After several years of denying that she had taken performance-enhancing drugs, Jones admitted to using steroids when she had competed in the 2000 Olympics in Sydney, Australia. At her trial she was convicted of lying to federal agents about the drug use and sentenced to 6 months in prison followed by 2 years of probation and 800 hours of community service. In addition, the International Olympic Committee stripped her of the 3 gold and 2 bronze medals that she had won and wiped her name and record-beating competition times from the record books. During a press conference Jones apologized profusely to her family, her friends, and her fans.

After her release from prison, Jones spoke on television about what she had done and how she felt about being sentenced to prison. She said:

I believe in the legal system . . . and I didn't want to go. Sure, I can compare my story to recent stories about other athletes or other people who were involved in certain situations and didn't get much time. It would be easy to do that. It would be easy to point the finger and say, "It's the judge." But you know what? It's me. I made the bad choice to put my future and my freedom in somebody else's hands to make that choice for me. I did that. And because of that, I have to live with it.[1]

Performance-Enhancing Drugs

The drugs that are used most often by athletes are anabolic or anabolic-androgenic steroids. The word *anabolic* refers to a steroid's ability to help build muscle, while *androgenic* refers to the drug's role in promoting the development of male sexual characteristics. Steroids, which may be taken orally or injected, cause muscles to grow faster, increase muscle mass, and increase strength, thereby boosting athletic performance. These steroids are made in a laboratory and are synthetic forms of testosterone, the naturally produced male hormone. According to the Drug Enforcement Administration (DEA), there are more than 100 different types of anabolic steroids.

Another way athletes attempt to boost their sports performance is to use synthetic forms of human growth hormone (HGH). In the human body HGH is produced naturally by the pituitary gland, which is located at the base of the brain and stimulates the growth of muscle, cartilage, and bone. Athletes inject high doses of synthetic HGH in an effort to increase muscle size, gain strength and stamina, and increase speed—but whether the drug actually works has been questioned. In a March 24, 2007, article, *Slate* senior editor Daniel Engber discussed this. "What's the difference between

> " Steroids, which may be taken orally or injected, cause muscles to grow faster, increase muscle mass, and increase strength, thereby boosting athletic performance. "

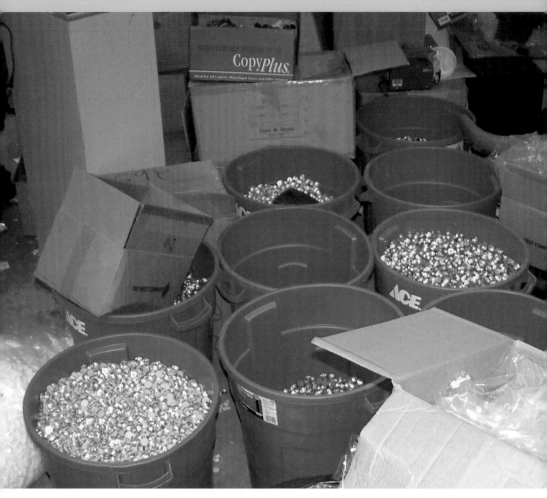

Buckets brimming with steroids confiscated in 2007 are displayed after an 18-month international investigation that led to more than 120 arrests and the seizure of 56 U.S. manufacturing laboratories. Many sports have been stung by reports of athletes using steroids and other performance-enhancing drugs.

steroids and HGH?" he asked. "For starters, we know that a baseball player can beef up on steroids and improve his athletic performance. But most clinical studies suggest that HGH won't help an athlete at all."[2] A study published in June 2007 by the Garvan Institute in Sydney, Australia, confirmed Engber's perspective. The researchers found that HGH had no effect on muscle mass or sports performance, and the increased weight gain experienced by some who take the drug is likely due to excess fluid retention.

Illicit Drugs

In addition to performance-enhancing drugs, athletes have also been caught using drugs that are banned under federal law, such as marijuana, cocaine, and methamphetamine. Stories of drug problems abound, touching prominent professional athletes in sports ranging from football, basketball, and baseball to tennis, hockey, and swimming.

In May 2009 NASCAR driver Jeremy Mayfield tested positive for methamphetamine. Although Mayfield denied taking the drug, insisting that the positive test was due to a mixture of over-the-counter allergy medication and a prescription drug, NASCAR suspended him indefinitely. He was the first driver to be suspended under the organization's new drug-testing policy for 2009 that mandates pre-season testing for drivers, crew members, and series officials and also allows for random testing during the racing season. In spite of the suspension, however, Mayfield's sentence was later overturned by a federal judge, who said that NASCAR's drug-testing system was flawed. But in July, after he tested positive for methamphetamine a second time, a federal appeals court ruled in NASCAR's favor and reinstated Mayfield's suspension.

> " **Anyone caught using steroids for nonmedical reasons, such as to enhance athletic performance, is doing so illegally and is subject to arrest and punishment if caught.** "

A number of other athletes have also been caught using illicit drugs. One was Olympic swimmer Michael Phelps, who has won more gold medals than any other athlete in history. After a photograph surfaced in 2009 showing Phelps smoking marijuana, he apologized, saying that he had exercised bad judgment by using the drug.

What the Law Says About Performance-Enhancing Drugs

One of the most obvious reasons many people object to athletes using performance-enhancing drugs is that they are often obtained illegally and/or used for nonmedical reasons. Since 1991 the DEA had listed anabolic steroids as a controlled substance under the Controlled Substances Act, meaning that they can only legally be prescribed by physicians for medical conditions. For instance, steroids may be prescribed for men who have lower-than-normal levels of testosterone, as well as for people who have diseases that result in the wasting of muscle mass.

Anyone caught using steroids for purposes such as increasing muscle mass or enhancing athletic performance is doing so illegally and is subject to arrest and punishment if caught. The same is true with HGH, which is also available through prescription. HGH is used to treat conditions such as growth hormone deficiency and chronic kidney disease, and it can also help injured muscles heal faster. But as with steroids, athletes may abuse HGH by using it to enhance sports performance rather than for medical reasons.

How Serious a Problem Is Drug Use Among Athletes?

It is impossible to determine with any certainty how many athletes use drugs because there is no way to know how many do so and are not caught. Yet athletes who participate in all types of sports have tested positive for banned drugs such as steroids. This has proved to be especially true in professional sports. A June 2007 report by former senator George Mitchell revealed that performance-enhancing drug use has been widespread among Major League Baseball players, and the report identified more than 80 players as users. There have also been documented reports of professional basketball players using drugs. And according to a June 2008 article by physicians Michael F. Schafer and Mary Ann Porucznik, "[Performance-enhancing drug] use has also been documented among Olympic athletes, weightlifters, football players, NASCAR drivers, and competitive cyclists."[3]

> "One reason it is difficult to determine the seriousness of drug use among athletes is that not all drugs are detectable through testing."

In recent years competitive cycling has seen its share of publicity over performance-enhancing drugs, especially among competitors in the annual Tour de France. The Tour is a grueling bicycle race that lasts 3 weeks and takes riders over approximately 2,200 miles (3,500km) in and around France. Between 2005 and 2008 numerous participants tested positive for performance-enhancing drugs, which caused the International Cycling Union to toughen its drug-testing program. During the race a minimum of 4 teams per day are now subject to random drug testing. Also, all finishers are tested after every stage of the race, as are other riders who are selected at random.

Drug use is not confined to Olympic athletes or those who play professional sports. There have also been numerous cases of drug use among athletes at the college level. Drew Johnson played on the baseball team at Thomas University in Thomasville, Georgia. During his freshman year, he says, 13 of his teammates took steroids. Johnson refused to use the drugs, and he believes that doing so gives players an unfair edge. "So that was 13 spots that were taken up and here I was doing the right thing," he says. "But all these guys were getting playing time ahead of me. It wasn't fair to me."[4] High school students have also admitted to using performance-enhancing drugs. A December 2008 report by the National Institute on Drug Abuse showed that 1.4 percent of eighth graders, 1.4 percent of tenth graders, and 2.2 percent of twelfth graders have used steroids at least once.

One reason it is difficult to determine the seriousness of drug use among athletes is that not all drugs are detectable through testing. For instance, if an athlete has taken steroids, the drugs almost always show up during commercially available urine tests. But the same is not true of HGH. Synthetic HGH looks identical to the natural hormone and has the same sequence of amino acids, so it cannot be detected through urine testing. Some blood tests can detect HGH, but they are often not given to athletes because the tests must be performed within 48 hours of the drug being used. Also, blood tests are a source of controversy because

> **Throughout the entire year, at unannounced times and in various places where athletes live, train, and/or compete, all Olympians must be prepared to provide two urine samples.**

they are considered invasive. Thus, it is probable that most athletes who use HGH to enhance sports performance are never found out.

Influence on Teen Athletes

People who denounce professional athletes for using performance-enhancing drugs say that this will inevitably lead to widespread use among young athletes who see these sports stars as heroes and role models. As Mitchell stated in his December 2007 report:

> Apart from the dangers posed to the major league player himself . . . his use of performance enhancing substances encourages young athletes to use those substances. Young Americans are placing themselves at risk of serious harm. Because adolescents are already subject to significant hormonal changes, the abuse of steroids and other performance enhancing substances can have more serious effects on them than they have on adults.

Mitchell added that estimates seem to indicate a decline in steroid use by high school students, ranging from 3 to 6 percent. "But, he said, "even the lower figure means that hundreds of thousands of high school–aged young people are still illegally using steroids."[5]

> Although the NCAA is the governing body for sports played at colleges and universities throughout the United States, the organization leaves most drug-testing decisions to its members.

Reports about how many young athletes are influenced to take drugs often vary. According to a 2008 poll of teenagers by *Sports Illustrated*, 99 percent of respondents said they would not use steroids just because a professional athlete does. Other studies, however, have netted different results, with more teenagers admitting that they had taken steroids specifically to enhance athletic performance. For example, a 2005 National Youth Risk Behavior Survey showed that 4 percent of high school students admitted using illegal steroids, down from 6.1 percent in 2003.

But a later survey showed that 6 percent of twelfth-grade males reported using steroids, of whom 80 percent believed the drugs could help them achieve their athletic dreams.

Drug Policies for Olympic and Professional Athletes

The Olympics organization has a tough, no-tolerance drug code for its athletes. Overseen in the United States by the U.S. Anti-Doping Agency and globally by the World Anti-Doping Agency (WADA), the policy

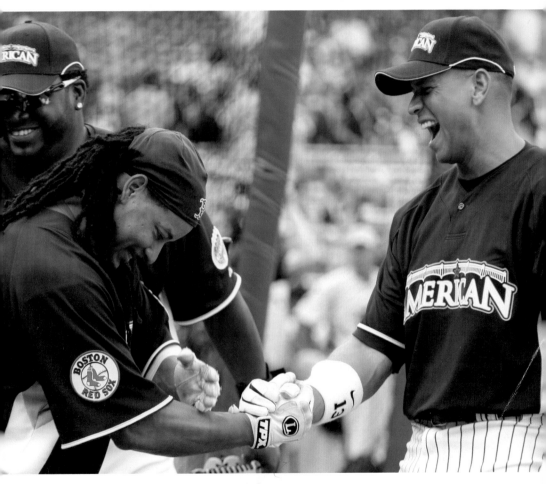

Three of baseball's top players, (from left) David Ortiz, Manny Ramirez, and Alex Rodriguez, greet each other during 2008 All-Star batting practice. All three have recently been linked to performance-enhancing substances or steroids.

provides a list of banned substances, including steroids, stimulants, and hormones. Throughout the entire year, at unannounced times and in various places where athletes live, train, and/or compete, all Olympians must be prepared to provide two urine samples. If the first tests positive, the athlete may be banned from taking part in competitions until the second sample has been tested. If it also tests positive, the International Olympic Committee may strip the athlete of any medals that have been won and ban him or her from taking part in the games for a specified period of a time, including for life.

Unlike the Olympic drug-testing policy, which is consistent for all athletes who compete, professional sports associations have their own rules about drugs and drug testing. For example, the National Hockey League randomly tests players up to 3 times per year during hockey season, with the exception of playoffs. The National Football League (NFL) tests all players at least once during football season; and randomly selects players to be tested during the off-season. NASCAR's policy calls for random tests of 2 samples from 8 to 15 drivers and crew members each week during racing season. The Professional Golfers' Association never had a drug or drug-testing policy in the past, as it believed such policies were unnecessary. As of 2008, however, the association can test any golfer at any time or place, during or out of competition, without advance notice.

Drug-Testing Policies in Schools

Drug-testing policies at American high schools often differ from institution to institution. Currently, only New Jersey, Texas, and Illinois have adopted statewide random steroid screening programs in order to prevent the use of performance-enhancing drugs among high school athletes. New Jersey's policy, which was the first in the country, involves testing 240,000 athletes through a private agency hired by the New Jersey Interscholastic Athletic Association. Bob Baly, the assistant director of the state's athletic association, explains the reasoning behind the effort: "I want kids to think that there's a cop at the end of the corner, so they don't speed."[6] Most states, however, do not have such legislation in place. Florida implemented a drug-testing program in 2004 but abandoned it 4 years later because only 1 athlete out of 600 students tested positive. Three other states, Delaware, Louisiana, and California, have considered and rejected steroid testing at the high school level.

Drug testing of college athletes is overseen by the National Collegiate Athletic Association (NCAA). The agency partners with the National Center for Drug Free Sport to test all divisions of its athletes at team and individual championships. According to a March 2008 article in *Sports Illustrated*, college athletes can be selected randomly for testing at all rounds of NCAA championship events. The article adds that the punishment for a positive test is a one-year ban on athletic participation, and a second positive tests means the athlete loses NCAA eligibility. For some sports, athletes may also be subjected to out-of-season testing.

How Effective Are Drug-Testing Policies?

Most professional sports organizations have drug-testing policies, although the stringency of the policies often varies. The people who support the toughest drug-testing programs say that professional athletes should have to abide by the same tough rules as Olympic athletes. But unlike the Olympics, there is no umbrella law or entity that mandates drug testing for professional athletes. Instead, each sports organization has its own testing and punishment policies, and some people are convinced that should change. They believe there should be legislation that would make professional sports organizations implement tougher, more uniform drug-testing policies that demand at least five surprise drug tests on every athlete per year, as well as stiffer penalties for athletes who violate drug policies.

Those who oppose mandatory drug testing for athletes say that such tests violate the Constitution's Fourth Amendment, which prohibits unreasonable search or seizure without probable cause. This is the perspective of the Women's Sports Foundation, which writes: "The Foundation is against any unreasonable invasion of privacy and believes that drug testing is an intrusion into the physical person that constitutes unreasonable

> **Those who oppose mandatory drug testing for athletes say that such tests violate the Constitution's Fourth Amendment, which prohibits unreasonable search or seizure without probable cause.**

search when drug testing is conducted without cause." The group adds, though, that the pressure to win in competitive sports means that drug use is likely among elite athletes. "Therefore, the Foundation supports impartially administered, unannounced random and voluntary drug testing programs conducted according to protocols that eliminate the possibility of error and protect the rights of athletes and their coaches."[7]

Is More Rigorous Drug Testing Needed for Student Athletes?

Whether high school and college athletes should be subjected to tougher drug-testing rules is a controversial issue. Many people are convinced that such testing is necessary in order to deter student athletes from using drugs. Others disagree, saying that mandatory testing is inappropriate, especially at the high school level. That is the perspective of Howard Jacobs, a defense attorney who specializes in drug-related issues. Jacobs refutes the idea that high school drug-testing programs should mirror what is done with Olympic athletes: "The logic in the Olympics is that this is your job and it's reasonable to expect that you'll subject yourself to extremely rigorous testing. How do you apply that to a ninth-grade varsity soccer player? It's just not appropriate to bring Olympic-quality testing to high schools."[8]

Controversy also exists over whether colleges should implement more rigorous drug-testing policies for athletes. Although the NCAA is the governing body for sports played at colleges and universities throughout the United States, the organization leaves most drug-testing decisions to its members. They are allowed to set their own policies about what substances they test for, how often testing takes place, and how to punish those who test positive. They are even able to make independent decisions about whether to test athletes at all. As a result, there is vast disparity from one school to another.

Should Drug Use Be Legalized in Competitive Sports?

Even with all the public denouncements of sports-enhancing drug use by professional athletes, this is a hotly debated topic. Just as passionate as those who want such practices stopped are others who argue that these drugs should be legal. As a June 2009 editorial in the *New York Times* states: "The purists' last argument is that players' use of performance-enhancing drugs sets a bad example for young athletes. But baseball players aren't children; they are adults in a very stressful and competitive profession. If they want to use anabolic steroids, or human growth hormone or bull's testosterone, it should be up to them."[9] People who disagree with that perspective say that performance-enhancing drugs should remain illegal because they give athletes an unfair edge over others who choose not to take the drugs. Another argument is that the potential side effects can endanger athletes' health.

A Difficult Problem to Solve

Drug use by athletes is an issue that is fraught with controversy. Many people are adamantly against any drugs in sports and push for tougher drug policies and stricter penalties for violators. Others argue against mandatory testing at any level, from high school to professional sports. Some even advocate for the legalization of performance-enhancing drugs, saying that professional and Olympic athletes should have the freedom to choose for themselves whether to use the drugs. Because of the strong, vastly different opinions on all sides of this issue, it is not likely to be resolved anytime soon.

How Serious a Problem Is Drug Use Among Athletes?

66Professional and amateur sports are awash in steroids and have been for many years. It seems self-evident that this is a problem.99

—Arthur Caplan, director of the Center for Bioethics at the University of Pennsylvania.

66As we've argued, performance enhancement is not against the spirit of sport, it's been a part of sport through its whole history, and to be human is to be better, or at least to try to be better.99

—Julian Savulescu, professor of practical ethics at the University of Oxford.

Prior to the 1970s there were no policies or rules that governed the use of performance-enhancing drugs, either for Olympians or professional athletes. In fact, in 1963 the San Diego Chargers won the American Football League championship game, and it was later revealed that the coach had given all the players daily doses of steroids throughout their entire time at training camp. This did not result in much controversy, though, because steroids were not prohibited. Public awareness and concern about athletes' use of performance-enhancing drugs began to grow after *Sports Illustrated* published the first investigative series about the issue in 1969. It focused on the seriousness of drug use among professional athletes and exposed how widespread the problem was. Publisher

Gary Valk introduced the series by calling drug use in sport a "vastly complicated problem" and added that there was "astonishingly wide use" of drugs by athletes. "It is a problem that many of the rulers of sport pretend does not exist," Valk wrote, "in the misguided hope that it will go away. We do not believe it will vanish of its own accord."[10]

In the decades since the publication of the *Sports Illustrated* series, most professional sports organizations, as well as the International Olympic Committee, the NCAA, and a number of high school sports groups have banned performance-enhancing drugs, along with numerous other drugs. In spite of the bans, drug use among athletes has continued. Even with tough drug policies and random testing, drugs have been shown to be very much a part of all types of sports, at all levels.

Perspectives on Performance-Enhancing Drugs

Many people object to performance-enhancing drugs because they think athletes who use them are cheating. Steroids are known for increasing muscle mass and speed, and those who oppose them say that this gives users an unfair advantage over athletes who do not use drugs. Jim Bunning, a U.S. senator who was formerly a star pitcher with the Detroit Tigers, feels strongly that steroids have no place in professional sports. He is especially concerned because of the effect this can have on young people who idolize professional athletes. "If players who cheat to gain entrance into baseball's most elite club are given a free pass," Bunning writes, "it sends a terrible message to our nation's young athletes that it is OK to cheat." He adds that kids should be taught to work hard for something they want badly, rather than cheating to get it. "There are no shortcuts in life," he says. "But kids see home runs blasted like cannons and they want to feel that thrill and accomplish that feat for themselves. So they emulate these professional athletes any way they can. The competition in junior high and high school sports is tough and too many kids take the route of the needle and pill to get any edge they can over their opponents."[11]

> **Many people object to performance-enhancing drugs because they think athletes who use them are cheating.**

Although few would argue in favor of young athletes taking performance-enhancing drugs, many feel differently about professional and Olympic athletes. Some consider performance-enhancing drugs to be just one more way to build up one's body and gain a competitive advantage. This is the opinion of Steve Lyons, who is also a former Major League Baseball player. "Every day there's more speculation on who might be using performance enhancing drugs or who will be the next to be outted for their use," Lyons writes. "Why does anybody care how a ballplayer gets himself ready to play? Who does it really affect—except maybe himself?" According to Lyons, players have broken the rules in baseball since the game has existed by scuffing balls, corking bats, and sharpening cleats, practices that he says still take place today. Lyons is convinced that performance-enhancing drugs are no different. "So if you're beside yourself with disgust over the players that you think are using [performance-enhancing drugs] in today's game, get over it," he says. "It's just the latest way to try to get the advantage over the other guy."[12]

Illicit Drug Use

Studies have shown that athletes who participate in sports at all levels, from high school to professional, have tested positive for illicit drugs such as marijuana, cocaine, and methamphetamine, all of which are illegal in the United States. For instance, a study published in January 2008 by the National Collegiate Athletic Association revealed that a significantly higher number of college athletes tested positive for marijuana and other street drugs than for performance-enhancing drugs. At the professional level, one athlete who was caught with cocaine in his system is Tom Boonen, a top cyclist from Belgium. In April 2009 Boonen was suspended from participating in the Tour de France bicycle race after testing positive for the second time in a year.

Unknown Numbers

When famous professional sport stars admit to taking drugs, their stories are widely publicized by the media. For instance, in February 2009 New York Yankees baseball slugger Alex Rodriguez admitted that he had taken steroids from 2001 to 2003. But for every athlete like Rodriguez who is caught, there are undoubtedly many more who take drugs and do *not* get caught. This is especially true of HGH because it cannot be detected through urine tests, and players, along with their unions, often object to blood tests. As a result, there is no way to know with any accuracy how many professional athletes take drugs or how serious the drug problem actually is.

This is also the case with Olympic athletes. Anthony Butch, the director at the Olympic Analytical Laboratory at the University of California at Los Angeles, was asked by a reporter whether the International Olympic Committee is "winning the game" against athletes who use drugs. "It's impossible to answer," he said. "The reason we know we are making strides is we are catching more people, but to catch them, you have to know what they're abusing. It's possible there is something out there that everyone is taking that's not on the radar screens of the doping labs. We are always behind. It is easier to take these things and get away with it than it is to figure out ways to catch them."[13]

Nor is an exact number of college athletes who use performance-enhancing drugs known, although many suspect that drug use is prolific in collegiate sports. One instance occurred at the University of North Texas, where 86 football players were tested for drugs between September 24 and October 15, 2008. Fifteen players, or 17 percent, tested positive for drugs. That same year it was revealed that there is widespread use of drugs by college cheerleaders. In her book *Cheer! Three Teams on a Quest for College Cheerleading's Ultimate Prize*, author Kate Torgovnick reveals that male cheerleaders take steroids to build muscle so they are able to lift female cheerleaders into the air. Since the NCAA rates cheerleading as an activity rather than a sport, cheerleaders who take drugs are not often caught because they are not required to be tested.

Because so many high schools throughout the United States do not have drug-testing policies, knowledge of drug use among these athletes is especially cloudy. As a December 2007 *New York Daily News* article states: "Getting a reliable read on the number of teenage users of performance-enhancing drugs is about as easy as counting fish in the

> " **Even with tough drug policies and random testing, drugs have been shown to be very much a part of all types of sports, at all levels.** "

ocean." The article cites a youth behavior survey by the Centers for Disease Control and Prevention that found nearly 5 percent of twelfth-grade males had taken illegal steroids one or more times in their lives. "There are an estimated 14 million high school students in the country. If even 5% of them have taken illegal anabolic steroids, it puts the number of teenage users at 700,000."[14] Also of note is that high school drug use is largely gauged by surveys that the athletes fill out themselves, which means there is a strong possibility the numbers will not be accurate. Some sports officials say that student athletes may be reluctant to share information about their use of drugs, even in anonymous surveys.

The Dangers of Performance-Enhancing Drugs

When people discuss the seriousness of drug use among athletes, they often refer to the potential health risks. For example, when steroids are used regularly to increase muscle mass and strength, this can lead to a number of physical problems. The National Institute on Drug Abuse states that the major side effects include liver and kidney damage, cancer, and high blood pressure. The Drug Enforcement Administration (DEA) says that steroid abuse has been associated with cardiovascular disease, including heart attacks and strokes—even in athletes younger than 30. The DEA adds that steroids also increase the risk that blood clots will form in blood vessels, which could potentially disrupt blood flow and damage the heart.

> **Because so many high schools throughout the United States do not have drug-testing policies, knowledge of drug use among these athletes is especially cloudy.**

Another side effect associated with steroids is the development of severe acne on the body. In August 2008 dermatologists in Dusseldorf, Germany, were shocked when they examined a 21-year-old amateur bodybuilder who was taking high doses of steroids every day. The young man had developed a horrific case of acne that covered his upper back, chest, shoulders, and upper arms with abscesses and open wounds. The doctors convinced him to stop taking steroids and gave him medicines to kill the microorganisms that were causing the acne.

The skin disease disappeared within six weeks—and so did his muscle mass. He was left with a flabby upper body that was terribly scarred, and his doctors doubted whether he would ever be able to train again. One of his physicians, Peter Arne Gerber, explains: "It is questionable whether he will be able to start building muscle mass again—he may not be able to perform the exercises due to the scarring."[15]

> **Olympic athletes who are caught using banned substances are stripped of their medals and disallowed from competing again, and they also endure public humiliation for tarnishing their country's image.**

HGH abuse also poses serious risks to a user's health. According to Alan D. Rogol, who is a professor of pediatrics at the University of Virginia and at the Indiana University School of Medicine, high doses of HGH can cause acromegaly, a serious disease that can lead to severe muscle weakness and heart problems. "There are a number of FDA-approved uses of growth hormone in children and adults," Rogol states. "These do not include anti-aging or 'improvement' in athletic performance. The larger the doses of growth hormone administered the more [likely] moderate and serious side effects may occur."[16]

Punishments for Athletes Who Use Drugs

Those who view drug use in sports as a major problem say that athletes who test positive should be severely punished. Whether this happens as often as it should largely depends on the sport, as well as personal opinion. Olympic athletes who are caught using banned substances are stripped of their medals and disallowed from competing again, and they also endure public humiliation for tarnishing their country's image. In professional sports the Professional Golfers' Association has one of the toughest policies: The first violation may result in the golfer being ineligible to play for one year, while a second violation could lead to a five-year suspension of playing privileges and fines of up to $500,000.

Yet some athletes get off much more easily than others. Famed

> **Since drug testing has existed, people who play sports have been caught using banned substances from marijuana and cocaine to performance-enhancing drugs.**

baseball slugger Manny Ramirez was suspended in May 2009 for 50 games after testing positive for steroids. The suspension cost Ramirez more than $7 million, which sounds like a severe punishment, but it is a small amount compared to his $25 million salary. As sports writer Bob Smizik writes: "That would appear to be a heavy fine but it is little more than pocket change for Ramirez, who, when his current contract is complete, will have earned close to $200 million playing baseball. Crazy guy that Ramirez is, he might have thought the risk was worth it. He'll take off a couple of months and come back and finish out his contract." Smizik adds that although he has never been a fan of zero tolerance, it may be needed in professional sports: "Something like one failed test and your career is over. If that's too tough, then allow teams to void the contracts of the guilty."[17]

Scale of the Problem Unknown

Since drug testing has existed, people who play sports have been caught using banned substances from marijuana and cocaine to performance-enhancing drugs. Studies have shown that this is a problem in professional sports, the Olympics, and among student athletes. The seriousness of the problem is not known because for all those who test positive, many more may escape getting caught. Whether this issue will ever be more clearly identified—as well as whether it is resolvable—remains a mystery.

How Serious a Problem Is Drug Use Among Athletes?

66 There is an epidemic of steroid use in this country that is quietly being shoved under the rug because parents, coaches, and school administrators refuse to face the fact that steroids are dangerous—and illegal—drugs. 99

—Jim Evans, "Adverse Side Effects of Steroids Are Real—and Often Fatal," *Los Angeles Examiner*, June 3, 2009. www.examiner.com.

Evans is an internationally recognized fitness consultant.

66 The number of deaths from playing professional football and college football are 50 to 100 times higher than even the wild exaggerations about steroids. More people have died playing baseball than have died of steroid use. 99

—Norman Fost, "Should We Accept Steroid Use in Sports?" National Public Radio, January 23, 2008. www.npr.org.

Fost is a professor of pediatrics and bioethics at the University of Wisconsin.

Bracketed quotes indicate conflicting positions.

* Editor's Note: While the definition of a primary source can be narrowly or broadly defined, for the purposes of Compact Research, a primary source consists of: 1) results of original research presented by an organization or researcher; 2) eyewitness accounts of events, personal experience, or work experience; 3) first-person editorials offering pundits' opinions; 4) government officials presenting political plans and/or policies; 5) representatives of organizations presenting testimony or policy.

❝Over the last few years the sports world has been rocked by one scandal after another as high profile celebrity athletes were publicly caught with their hand in the performance enhancing drug cookie jar.❞

—Roman Mica, "When It Comes to Performance Enhancing Drugs, What's the Dirtiest Sport Today?" *Los Angeles Examiner*, August 5, 2009. www.examiner.com.

Mica is an amateur Clydesdale triathlete who lives and races in Boulder, Colorado, and the author of *No, Seriously My Training Begins Tomorrow: The Everyman's Guide to IRONFIT Swimming, Cycling & Running*.

❝Steroids are dangerous and sometimes fatal. Yet, if some players use them, others will feel the pressure to use them as well, in order to compete.❞

—Thomas Sowell, "Say It Ain't So," *National Review*, December 14, 2007.

Sowell is a senior fellow at Stanford University's Hoover Institution.

❝In most sports, it is my belief that performance-enhancing drug use is the rule, not the exception.❞

—Kate Schmidt, "Just Say Yes to Steroids," *Oakland (CA) Tribune*, October 21, 2007. http://sportsanddrugs.procon.org.

Schmidt is a former U.S. Olympic javelin thrower.

❝Illegal drug use in baseball is a matter of individual choice, and as long as the cheaters are ahead of the testers—and it will always be thus—some players will be willing to take their chances. There's too much money to be made and too little time to make it.❞

—Jordan Kobritz, "PEDs in Baseball No Longer Selig's Fault," The Biz of Baseball, May 16, 2009. www.bizofbaseball.com.

Kobritz is a Business of Sports Network staff writer.

66 **The latest revelation of stars using chemicals to hit the ball farther and throw it harder was another blow to baseball.** 99

—Clark Hoyt, "Baseball's Top-Secret Roster," *New York Times*, August 8, 2009. www.nytimes.com.

Hoyt is a columnist for the *New York Times*.

66 **Sport is a contest in character, not in chemistry or pharmacology. Not only is doping dangerous to one's health, it blatantly violates the spirit of sport.** 99

—Gary Wadler, quoted in Jeff Z. Klein, "Dr. Gary Wadler of the World Anti-Doping Agency Gives His Answers to Your Questions," *New York Times*, June 27, 2008. http://olympics.blogs.nytimes.com.

Wadler is chair of the World Anti-Doping Agency's Prohibited List and Methods Committee.

66 **One of my favorite authors [is] Baltimore native H.L. Mencken, who I think would've had a good laugh at the hypocrisy, the posturing, and the moral prudery associated with the steroid controversy.** 99

—Radley Balko, "Should We Allow Performance Enhancing Drugs in Sports?" *Reason*, January 23, 2008. www.reason.com.

Balko is the senior editor for *Reason* magazine.

66 **The drug of choice in the NBA long has been the cannabis plant, which is an almost quaint, amusing reality, considering the rampant use of performance-enhancing drugs in the NFL, major league baseball, the Olympics and the Tour de France.** 99

—Tom Knott, "Like All Sports, NBA Is Past Going to Pot," *Washington Times*, August 12, 2009.

Knott is a columnist for the *Washington Times* newspaper.

How Serious a Problem Is Drug Use Among Athletes?

- Since the **Professional Golfers' Association** implemented its drug-testing policy in 2008, no player has tested positive for drugs.

- An October 2007 poll published in the *Journal of the International Society of Sports Nutrition* showed that as many as **3 million** Americans may have used steroids for nonmedical purposes.

- Since 2007 only one **National Hockey League** player has tested positive for a banned substance.

- Of the 21,579 drug tests conducted at the Summer Olympics from 1968 to 2008, there were **59 cases** (0.27 percent) of drug violations.

- According to a survey published in 2009, nearly **1 in 10** retired National Football League players said they had used now-banned anabolic steroids while they were still playing.

- According to a study published in 2008, among students in grades 8 to 12 who admitted to using anabolic steroids, **57 percent** said professional athletes influenced their decision to use the drugs, and **63 percent** said pro athletes influenced their friends' decision to use drugs.

- In a poll of mixed martial arts fighters that was published in April 2009, **91.7 percent** of respondents admitted to using performance-enhancing drugs, and **79.3 percent** have used steroids to increase muscle mass and size.

Americans Are Concerned About Steroid Use

In a February 2009 poll by CBS News and the *New York Times*, participants were asked about their perceptions of Major League Baseball players using steroids. Nearly 90 percent of respondents had at least some concern about use of the drugs.

Question: *How much does it matter to you as a baseball fan if professional players use steroids or other performance-enhancing drugs? Do you care a lot, a little, or not at all?*

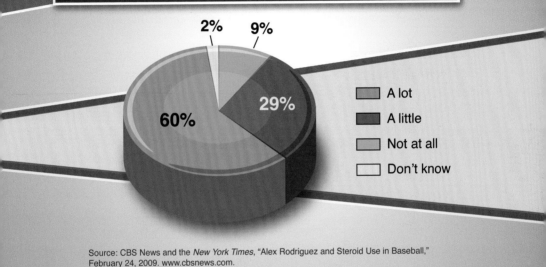

2% 9% 29% 60%

- A lot
- A little
- Not at all
- Don't know

Source: CBS News and the *New York Times*, "Alex Rodriguez and Steroid Use in Baseball," February 24, 2009. www.cbsnews.com.

- The North American Society for Sports Management states that the prevalence of steroid use has remained relatively stable over the last three decades, with approximately **2 to 3 percent** of twelfth-grade students reporting use of anabolic steroids.

- Studies have shown that the percentage of twelfth-grade students associating "great risk" with using steroids dropped from a high of **70.7 percent** in 1992 to **57.4 percent** in 2007.

Teenage Use of Steroids Versus Other Drugs

In May 2009 researchers from the University of Michigan's Institute for Social Research released a report called *Monitoring the Future: National Results on Adolescent Drug Use*. The report showed prevalence of drug use among high school students, finding that steroids are used far less than other drugs.

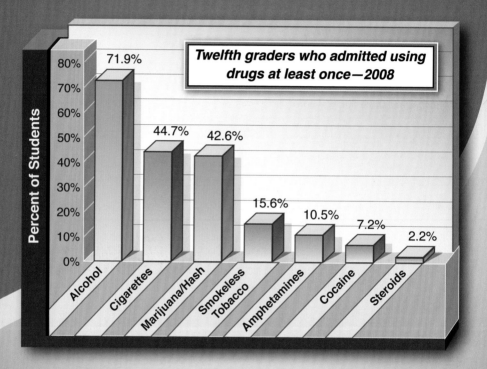

Source: Lloyd D. Johnston et al., *Monitoring the Future: National Results on Adolescent Drug Use*, May 2009. http://monitoringthefuture.org.

- The U.S. Department of Justice states that individuals who abuse steroids may take doses that are **10 to 100 times higher** than those used for medical conditions.

- According to the National Institute on Drug Abuse, steroid abuse is **higher among males** than females but is **growing most rapidly among young women**.

Public Perceptions About Drug Use by Olympic Athletes

Participants in a July 2008 *USA Today*/Gallup poll were asked to share their thoughts about the prevalence of performance-enhancing drugs in five of the most popular summer Olympic sports. The poll showed that fans perceive drug use as common in weightlifting but much less so in the other sports.

Question: *We'd like to know your views on how widespread the use of performance-enhancing drugs is in various Olympic sports. Just your best guess, how many Olympic athletes in weightlifting, track and field, cycling, swimming, and gymnastics use performance-enhancing drugs—all, most, some, only a few, or none?*

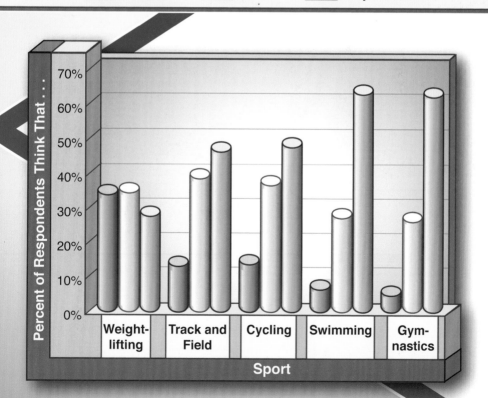

■ All/Most　　■ Some　　■ Only a few/None

Source: Jeffrey M. Jones, "Sports Fans Not Suspicious of Steroid Use for Record Breakers," Gallup, August 8, 2008. www.gallup.com.

Potential Side Effects of Steroids in Men and Women

Steroids are synthetic substances that are related to the male hormone testosterone. Many athletes use steroids to build muscle and improve speed and agility, but according to the National Institute on Drug Abuse, abuse of these drugs can result in a number of unwanted and even dangerous side effects.

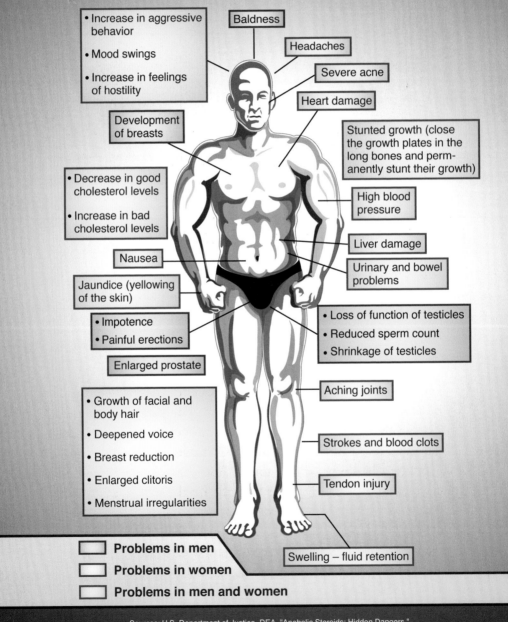

- Increase in aggressive behavior
- Mood swings
- Increase in feelings of hostility

Baldness

Headaches

Severe acne

Heart damage

Development of breasts

Stunted growth (close the growth plates in the long bones and permanently stunt their growth)

- Decrease in good cholesterol levels
- Increase in bad cholesterol levels

High blood pressure

Nausea

Liver damage

Jaundice (yellowing of the skin)

Urinary and bowel problems

- Impotence
- Painful erections

- Loss of function of testicles
- Reduced sperm count
- Shrinkage of testicles

Enlarged prostate

Aching joints

- Growth of facial and body hair
- Deepened voice
- Breast reduction
- Enlarged clitoris
- Menstrual irregularities

Strokes and blood clots

Tendon injury

☐ **Problems in men**

☐ **Problems in women**

☐ **Problems in men and women**

Swelling – fluid retention

Sources: U.S. Department of Justice, DEA, "Anabolic Steroids: Hidden Dangers," March 2008; *USA Today*, "How Anabolic Steroids Work," www.usatoday.com.

How Effective Are Drug-Testing Policies?

66It is a privilege to compete in athletics on the world stage: If an athlete doesn't like someone showing up at their door and can't handle a tester watching them provide a urine sample, then they can quit.99

—Nathan Jendrick, author, celebrity personal trainer, and fitness specialist.

66NASCAR's policy and procedures fall below those of baseball, football, basketball and even hockey, the latter of which offers a testing program with the teeth of a worm.99

—Ed Graney, sports columnist for the *Las Vegas Review-Journal*.

Whether sports drug-testing policies are as effective as they should be is a topic that is often debated. One point of contention is that professional sports organizations have drug-testing policies that are far more lenient than those of the Olympics, and many people think the policies should be equally tough. Also controversial is the fact that professional sports organizations have the freedom to set their own policies, some of which are perceived to be vague and ineffective. This was brought to light in July 2009, after NASCAR driver Jeremy Mayfield tested positive for methamphetamine. Although officials use an independent company to administer drug testing, the final decisions about punishment are left up to the NASCAR organization.

According to officials from the World Anti-Doping Agency (WADA) and the U.S. Anti-Doping Agency, NASCAR does not have an effective drug policy in place. They claim that punishment guidelines are not clearly spelled out, nor are drivers given a list of banned substances. This ambiguity is what led to Mayfield's drug suspension being overturned by a federal judge, who noted that NASCAR's drug-testing program was flawed. U.S. Anti-Doping Agency CEO Travis Tygart says that the Mayfield case "will be used as Exhibit 1 of what can go horribly wrong when you don't have an effective policy in place."[18] Tygart adds that testing programs for professional sports organizations need to have sanctions that are clearly spelled out, along with a distinct, fair process for those who are being punished. He speaks of the effect Mayfield's case could have on other drivers: "The truly clean drivers, frankly, should be outraged. Because you either have a drug user who got off on a technicality due to poor policy, or you have a clean athlete who is falsely accused. Either way, I'd be scared to death if I were a driver."[19] Mayfield's suspension was later reinstated, however, when he tested positive a second time and a federal appeals court ruled in NASCAR's favor.

> "One point of contention is that professional sports organizations have drug-testing policies that are far more lenient than those of the Olympics, and many people think the policies should be equally tough."

Proposed Legislation

At a congressional hearing in February 2008, sports officials and members of Congress discussed drug-testing policies of the major professional sports organizations. They were revisiting the issue of whether drug testing should remain as is, with the various organizations setting their own policies, or be mandated by federal law. The hearing was largely the result of an investigative report by former senator George Mitchell that revealed widespread steroid problems among professional baseball players. Mitchell strongly supports federal drug-testing policies for professional sports organizations similar to those used in Olympic sports. Under the proposed legislation, the federal government would impose standard testing and punishment requirements on all professional sports leagues.

No progress was made toward implementing such a law, however. Commissioners from Major League Baseball, the National Football League (NFL), the National Hockey League, and the National Basketball Association (NBA) strongly objected to what they perceived as one-size-fits-all regulations. They emphasized that their organizations' drug-testing policies should remain in place because they have proved to be effective over the years. Speaking at the February hearing, David Stern, commissioner of the NBA, said that federal legislation was not necessary because his organization and the others had "gotten it right" over the past three years. Tennessee congresswoman Marsha Blackburn disagreed. "Mr. Stern," she said, "I would suggest that we have not gotten it right enough. If we had gotten it right—if you all had gotten it right—we would not be here . . . today."[20]

In March 2009 Edwin Moses, a former Olympic gold medal winner in track and field, published an article denouncing the outcome of the congressional hearing, stating that "the politicians just pontificated and then sat back down." Moses, who often speaks publicly against athletes using drugs, criticized the current drug-testing system in professional sports. "I am pessimistic that anything will change," he writes. "Baseball is in a period of denial. To understand why, consider the contrast with amateur sports and the Olympics, where athletes must make themselves available for random drug tests by telling the governing bodies where they are going to be over a period of time." Moses adds that Olympic officials have shown their de-

> "Commissioners from Major League Baseball, the National Football League (NFL), the National Hockey League, and the National Basketball Association (NBA) strongly objected to what they perceived as one-size-fits-all regulations."

termination to fight drug use, and they back that up by banning athletes for up to two years for violations. "By contrast," he says, "professional sports merely attempts to 'manage the issue.'"[21]

Collective Bargaining and Drug Policies

Although many believe that professional sports organizations should have tougher, more consistent drug-testing policies, legislating those policies would not be an easy feat. U.S. labor laws dictate that drug-testing decisions are a part of the collective bargaining process, as Chicago attorney Lester Munson explains: "Any legislative proposal on testing and punishment would require a major change in American labor laws. Under current rules, which have been in place for generations, drug testing is a mandatory subject of collective bargaining. If the workers, including professional athletes, in any industry are covered by a union contract, the union and the industry management must agree on testing and on punishment."[22]

Because drug-testing policies are part of collective bargaining, some view this as a conflict of interest. In other words, professional athletes have a say in what sort of testing is imposed, as well as how violators should be punished—and that is controversial. Many sports officials realize this and are committed to having drug policies that are tough and consistent. Yet even when such policies are in place, they are sometimes challenged by the very athletes who agreed to them. This occurred during the 2008 football season, when two Minnesota Vikings players were suspended for four games after testing positive for a banned substance that is known for masking steroids. The players hired attorneys and appealed their suspensions based on state laws. According to NFL officials, even if state statutes could potentially excuse the two men, the laws are superseded by the drug policies that have been collectively bargained. This position was applauded by the U.S. Anti-Doping Agency, as well as officials from the other major professional sports organizations.

> **Because drug-testing policies are part of collective bargaining, some view this as a conflict of interest.**

Jeff Pash, general counsel for the NFL, expressed gratitude for the support that had been shown by people who sided with officials in suspending the players. "The leagues all have collective bargaining agreements and they have teams in Minnesota, and they understand the importance of having uniform testing programs that apply to all players," he says. "To say that players in Minnesota get an exemption makes no sense. It brings down the entire program." Pash adds that he appreciates the U.S. Anti-Doping Agency's perspective "that to preserve the integrity of the competition, and for fans to have confidence in the outcome, you have to have one set of rules."[23] In September 2009 a federal appeals court ruled in the players' favor, stating that they could both play for the entire season. Troubled by the ruling, NFL officials planned to pursue the matter further.

> " **WADA now requires Olympic athletes to be available 365 days a year, including weekends and holidays, as well as days when they are traveling or competing.** "

The Complexities of Drug Testing

Even sports organizations that have tough drug policies in place often face challenges involved with drug testing. According to Frank Uryasz, president of the National Center for Drug Free Sport, drug testing is highly complex. Drugs are constantly changing, growing numbers are available through online sales, and athletes are becoming more adept at figuring out how to outwit drug tests to avoid being caught. Uryasz says that this "win-at-all-cost attitude fuels an industry for the manufacture and sale of performance-enhancing products that entices even our youngest athletes." He adds that even the most seemingly ironclad drug-testing policy may be flawed: "The science involves measurement and all measurement has error. The science also includes probability and human interpretation. Strict laboratory protocols and redundancies in our systems reduce such error to levels of acceptability."[24]

To support his belief about the possibility of lab errors, Uryasz cites a 2007 study published by Harvard Medical School. Although the study was not specifically related to sports drug testing, its findings reveal the complexities of testing in general and the potential for human error. The researchers analyzed drug test results from more than 100 adolescent drug users and found that out of 710 drug tests, 85 were susceptible to error. The study's conclusion states: "Unless proper procedures are used in collecting, analyzing and interpreting the laboratory testing for drugs, there is a substantial risk for error."[25] In order to ensure that drug-testing programs are as effective as possible, Uryasz urges all sports organizations to assess carefully whether their drug policies have kept pace with the many complexities of drug use, including what substances players might use in an attempt to mask drug use when they are tested.

The Debate over Rigidity

The Olympics organization is widely respected for its drug policy, which is overseen in the United States by the U.S. Anti-Doping Agency and globally by WADA. The policy is strict, clearly spelled out, and easily understood. It is often hailed as the type of program that should govern all athletics, including professional sports. Yet in January 2009, when WADA's drug-testing policy became even more rigid, a number of people were frustrated and angry. Under previous rules, which were already viewed as the toughest of all sports organizations, athletes were required to keep Olympic officials apprised of their whereabouts at all times and to be available Monday through Friday (excluding holidays) for drug testing. To keep athletes informed about impending drug tests, they or their coaches or agents could be notified by telephone so they would know when a drug tester was going to visit them. The new policy, however, radically changed those rules.

WADA now requires Olympic athletes to be available 365 days a year, including weekends and holidays, as well as days when they are traveling or competing. They are required to set aside 1 hour every day, sometime from 6:00 A.M. to 11:00 P.M., for drug testing, and they must furnish this information 3 months in advance. And no longer can athletes find out ahead of time if they are going to be tested. The new rules forbid any advance notification whatsoever, so a drug tester can show up at an athlete's doorstep anytime during the year, any day of the week, during the predetermined hour. If athletes violate any of the rules, even unintentionally, it can lead to serious consequences. Missing 3 drug tests within an 18-month period during an athlete's appointed hour is interpreted as a positive drug test, and this can result in a 1- to 2-year ban from Olympic competition.

The new rules have sparked fierce protest from some Olympic athletes. After the new policy took effect, a group of British rowers sent a letter to WADA officials to explain their objections. They wrote:

> We have grave reservations about the principles underpinning the "Whereabouts" regime, and its implementation, and we feel that unless the system is changed, there will be a number of clean athletes facing life bans and a higher number of clean athletes who will opt to retire rather than face the constant hassle and panic of staying on top of these requirements, and the severe penalties for tripping up. Will this system catch more cheats, or merely compromise the lives and training of clean athletes? [26]

The rowers made it clear that the new policy was causing them anxiety and stress and was disrupting their lives. "We spend our days panicking; having to always think about when our nominated hour is on that day, any upcoming changes of plans, if there's any chance recently that we've missed a test. We absolutely support both no-notice testing and strict sanctions; what we object to is this impractical and unworkable regime. There are far better ways of catching doping cheats than this."[27]

The Debate Continues

People have differing opinions about mandatory drug testing for athletes. Those who believe such testing is necessary often point to the Olympics' policy, which is tough and consistent, although some athletes object to its rigidity. Most professional sports officials agree that testing should be mandatory for their athletes, but they want to make their own policies and object to legislation being imposed on them by the government. Then there are others who do not believe drug testing should be done at all. Can this be resolved? Because all who are involved feel equally passionate about their beliefs, a resolution that makes everybody happy is not likely to happen.

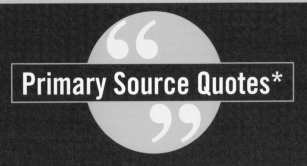

Primary Source Quotes*

How Effective Are Drug-Testing Policies?

"We need better testing, harsher punishments and people will decide not to get involved with performance-enhancing drugs."

—Dale Murphy, "Should We Accept Steroid Use in Sports?" National Public Radio, January 23, 2008. www.npr.org.

Murphy is a former Major League Baseball player who founded the antidrug group iWontCheat Foundation.

"Whether it's worth implementing any particular testing and enforcement regime has to take into account that the scheme is going to fail to some extent. Given the endless inventiveness of the human mind, the drug users will always be at least half a step ahead of the drug testers."

—Paul Campos, "Campos: Is Sports Drug War Worth It?" *Rocky Mountain News*, February 18, 2009. www.rockymountainnews.com.

Campos is a professor of law at the University of Colorado.

* Editor's Note: While the definition of a primary source can be narrowly or broadly defined, for the purposes of Compact Research, a primary source consists of: 1) results of original research presented by an organization or researcher; 2) eyewitness accounts of events, personal experience, or work experience; 3) first-person editorials offering pundits' opinions; 4) government officials presenting political plans and/or policies; 5) representatives of organizations presenting testimony or policy.

"The sporting public has been lied to so many times that we all just roll our eyes when an athlete tries to explain his way out of being busted for a failed drug test."

—Mike Bianchi, "Magic Forward Rashard Lewis Guilty of Stupidity, but Not of Drug Use," *Orlando Sentinel*, August 6, 2009. www.orlandosentinel.com.

Bianchi is sports columnist with the *Orlando Sentinel* newspaper.

"Fans, the media and sports governing bodies believe that we can rid sports of steroid use. Athletes always will be a step ahead of the testing labs in concealing substances because of the multibillion-dollar industries that have been built on their sweat and their obsession."

—Kate Schmidt, "Time to Legalize Steroids," *Dallas Morning News*, October 28, 2007. www.dallasnews.com.

Schmidt is a former U.S. Olympic javelin thrower.

"No drug testing program is perfect. The current drug testing program in Major League Baseball is the product of the give and take inherent in collective bargaining."

—George J. Mitchell, *Report to the Commissioner of Baseball of an Independent Investigation into the Illegal Use of Steroids and Other Performance Enhancing Substances by Players in Major League Baseball*, ESPN, December 13, 2007. http://assets.espn.go.com.

Mitchell is a former U.S. senator from Maine who investigated the use of performance-enhancing drugs among baseball players.

"If cricket shied away from a tough drug-testing regime, there's no guarantee doping wouldn't escalate and then down the track fans would have doubts, like there are in baseball now, over players' records."

—Ian Chappell, "The Price to Pay," *ESPNcricinfo*, August 2, 2009. www.cricinfo.com.

Chappell is a former captain of Australia's cricket team and is now a cricket commentator and columnist.

❝Can you blame us for being skeptical? They failed the tests! Doesn't that mean they cheated? Maybe, but for all the sports coverage on radio and television and in newspapers, we know little of how drug testing works, or if it does determine who uses prohibited drugs.❞

—Skip Rozin, "The Inside Dope: How Sports Drug Testing Works," *Wall Street Journal*, November 28, 2007. www.opinionjournal.com.

Rozin writes about sports-related subjects for the *Wall Street Journal*.

❝But here's the rub: call it freedom of contract if you like, but the unmistakable trend in drug testing agreements is that the leagues will test for so-called 'street' drugs such as cocaine or marijuana at the same time they test for steroids. Why does the decision to rid the games of performance enhancers necessarily include testing for marijuana?❞

—Jeffrey Standen, "Drug Testing Addiction," Sports Law Professor, January 26, 2007. http://thesportslawprofessor.blogspot.com.

Standen is a professor of law at the University of Virginia.

❝If you want to come (to Nevada) to fight, you are subject to testing. No one is forced to come here and fight. It's a privileged license.❞

—Keith Kizer, interviewed by Dann Stupp, "NSAC Executive Director Keith Kizer Discusses Year-Round Drug Testing," Mixed Martial Arts Junkie, January 30, 2008. http://mmajunkie.com.

Kizer is the executive director of the Nevada State Athletic Commission.

Facts and Illustrations

How Effective Are Drug-Testing Policies?

- Between 2001 and 2008 the total number of Olympic athletes tested for banned substances by the U.S. Anti-Doping Agency rose from **4,716 to nearly 7,700**.

- The **National Hockey League** randomly tests players up to three times per year during the hockey season with the exception of playoffs.

- The 2009 budget for the U.S. Anti-Doping Agency (which oversees Olympic athlete drug testing) is $13.3 million, with approximately **74 percent** from the federal government and **26 percent** from the U.S. Olympic Committee.

- NASCAR's drug-testing policy calls for random tests of two samples from **8 to 15 drivers and crew members** each week during racing season, although penalties are at the sole discretion of NASCAR officials.

- As of 2008 **professional golfers** may be tested by the Professional Golfers' Association at any time or place, during or out of competition, without advance notice.

- During the 2008 Olympics in Beijing, China, approximately **4,500 drug tests** were administered to athletes.

- The **National Football League** began testing for steroids in 1987 and started suspending violators in 1989 upon their first positive steroid test; a year-round random testing program has been in place since 1990.

The Expansion of Olympic Drug Testing

The Olympics Committee has thousands of chemical substances on its banned substance list and performs drug tests throughout the entire year, including when athletes are competing, training, and/or traveling. From 2001 the number of tests steadily rose until 2006 and then declined slightly over the next two years.

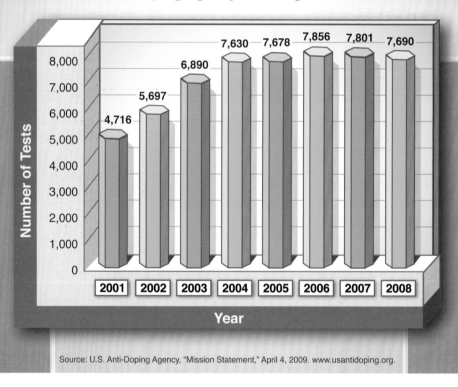

United States Anti-Doping Agency's Testing Numbers, 2001–2008

Source: U.S. Anti-Doping Agency, "Mission Statement," April 4, 2009. www.usantidoping.org.

- Under **Major League Baseball's** testing program, all **1,200 players** are tested for steroids and amphetamines within 5 days of arriving at spring training and are subject to at least 1 more test during the season, including the playoffs. Another 600 random tests are conducted, as many as 60 of them during the off-season.

Athletes' Views About Performance-Enhancing Drugs

Drug testing in most sports organizations discourages at least some athletes from taking performance-enhancing drugs because they do not want to risk getting caught. However, in a 2009 online poll of lacrosse players most of those surveyed said they would not take the drugs even if they knew they could get away with it.

If you knew you would never be caught and could be guaranteed it would make a huge difference in your game, would you take steroids during your career? Remember, no one would ever find out and your game would be taken to the next level every night out.

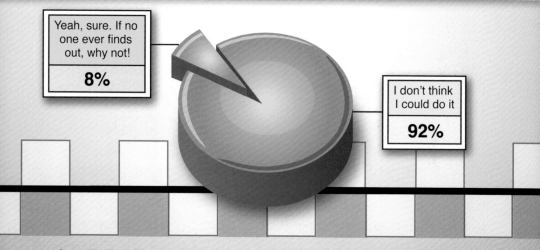

Yeah, sure. If no one ever finds out, why not!

8%

I don't think I could do it

92%

Source: Paul Tutka, "Player Poll: Steroid Use and Other Locker Room Taboos," NLL Insider, March 14, 2009. www.nllinsider.com.

- In 2007 **three** Major League Baseball players tested positive for steroids and were suspended for **50 games** each.

- Citing privacy violations, **65 athletes** from Belgium started court proceedings in 2009 to protest the Olympics rule that requires athletes to reveal their whereabouts 7 days a week, 365 days a year.

Vastly Different Drug Policies in Professional Sports

Most professional sports organizations have mandatory drug-testing policies in place, but those policies differ from sport to sport. In May 2008 ESPN published the results of a study that focused on performance-enhancing drug policies of six major professional sports, with all being measured against the tough policies of the Olympics Association.

Sports Organization	Drug Testing Policy	Punishment	ESPN Grade
NASCAR	Random tests of 8 to 15 drivers and crew members each week during racing season.	Penalties are at the sole discretion of NASCAR officials.	F
National Hockey League	Testing only during hockey season with the exception of play-offs; players are given advance notice that testers will arrive the next morning at practice.	First positive test: 20-game suspension.	D-
Professional Golfers' Association	Testing may be conducted at any time or place, during or outside of competition, without advance notice.	Policy states that sanctions "may" call for players to be suspended for 1 year after a first positive test, 5 years for a second, and permanently for a third; penalties are ultimately left up to the commissioner's discretion.	D-
National Basketball Association	Testing only during basketball season; players are subject to 4 tests per season, but samples are only collected at practices, game day shoot-arounds, or actual games.	First positive test: 10-day suspension, with 25 for a second.	D
National Football League	All players tested at least once during the season; each week 10 players from each team selected randomly to be tested, including off-season.	First positive test: 4-game suspension, with 8-game suspension for a second.	B
Major League Baseball	Tests for more drugs than any other sports organization; testing occurs throughout the year for all players, but only 10 percent are tested during off-season.	First positive test: 50-game suspension, 100 for the second, and a lifetime ban for the third.	B+

Source: Mark Fainaru-Wada and T.J. Quinn, "How U.S. Sports Measure Up to the 'Gold Standard' of Testing," ESPN, May 23, 2008. http://sports.espn.go.com.

Is More Rigorous Drug Testing Needed for Student Athletes?

> **For every argument advanced against random student drug testing, there are arguments in favor of such testing. . . . Even if random drug testing did not deter drug use, it still may be a useful tool to identify students using drugs at an early stage in order to allow intervention when it can be most effective.**
>
> —Supreme Court of the state of Washington, the highest court in the state.

> **The challenge is ferreting out the students using the drugs from those who are not. Random searches don't help. Why athletes and not the marching band or the cheerleading squad? And who monitors the students uninvolved in extracurricular activities?**
>
> —Editorial staff, *Seattle Times*, a major newspaper published in Seattle, Washington.

Drug testing is a controversial issue for many reasons, and at the heart of the debate is whether high school and college athletes should be subject to it. Those who see student drug testing as inappropriate and an invasion of privacy often cite the Fourth Amendment of the Constitution, which prohibits unreasonable search and seizure without probable cause. This claim was the gist of a case that was taken before the Supreme Court in 2002, *Board of Education of Independent*

School District No. 92 of Pottawatomie County v. Earls. Lindsay Earls and Daniel James, both students at Tecumseh High School in Oklahoma, objected to the school's policy of requiring drug tests before joining any extracurricular activity, as well as random testing while participating in the activity. Earls and James sued the school district, and after the U.S. district court rejected their claims, the Supreme Court agreed to hear the case.

> **The Office of National Drug Control Policy estimates that there are currently about 4,200 drug-testing programs at schools throughout the United States.**

In a June 27, 2002, decision, the majority of justices ruled in favor of the school district's drug-testing policy, with two caveats: that test results remain private and that school officials refrain from punishing students who test positive. Justice Clarence Thomas delivered the Court's opinion in a written statement. He addressed the concerns about constitutionality by stating: "Given the minimally intrusive nature of the sample collection and the limited uses to which the test results are put, we conclude that the invasion of students' privacy is not significant." Thomas stated the Court's opinion that testing students who participate in extracurricular activities was a "reasonably effective means of addressing the School District's legitimate concerns in preventing, deterring, and detecting drug use." His concluding statement summed up the ruling: "Evaluating the Policy in this context, we conclude that the drug testing of Tecumseh students who participate in extracurricular activities effectively serves the School District's interest in protecting the safety and health of its students."[28]

Expansion of Drug Testing in High Schools

After the Supreme Court ruling on the Tecumseh High School case, increasing numbers of schools throughout the United States began to implement drug-testing policies. In 2004 the federal government established funding for drug programs. Schools that were interested in implementing drug education and prevention programs, as well as drug-testing policies, were eligible for federal grants. According to a White House statement, as of 2009 the national drug control budget totaled $14.1 billion, of which $11.8 million was allocated for drug testing at schools. The Office of National Drug Control Policy estimates that there are currently about 4,200 drug-testing programs at schools throughout the United States, and the drugs that are included in the tests vary from program to program. For instance, in Cumberland County, North Carolina, all 12 high schools have drug-testing programs for athletes. Among the substances that the tests can detect are alcohol, marijuana, amphetamines, and performance-enhancing drugs.

Federal funding has helped some schools in Colorado implement drug-testing programs. Such testing is not mandatory on a statewide basis, but there has been growing interest in establishing programs at high schools for students who participate in sports, as well as other extracurricular activities such as 4-H and the debate team. During an April 2008 Random Student Drug Testing Summit in Pagosa Springs, Colorado, Harvard Medical School physician Bertha Madras urged administrators, teachers, coaches, and parents to implement random drug-testing policies at schools. She emphasized that such policies were the best tool to deter, identify, and treat drug use among students. "We are not waging a war on drugs," Madras told the group. "We are waging a war of defense—a defense of the basis of humanity, and that is our brain."[29]

> **Even though the NCAA has policies in place for colleges and universities throughout the United States, the organization does not dictate drug policies for individual schools.**

Yet along with growing support for Colorado's expanded school drug testing, there have also been strong objections. Those who oppose such policies see them as an erosion of individual rights and a dangerous expansion of government power. One who is against these policies for students is Cathryn Hazouri, who is the executive director of Colorado's American Civil Liberties Union. She explains: "I think the war on drugs is becoming a war on people. They are making the school into a watchdog, and that's more disruptive to the educational process than it is protective."[30]

This perspective was echoed in the state of Washington during 2008. The parents of three student athletes in Wahkiakum, Washington, sued the school district after their children were subjected to drug testing. The plaintiffs claimed that such testing, which was performed at the middle school and high school, was not supported by scientific research. They also said that the tests undermined the student-teacher relationship, could discourage students from participating in extracurricular activities, and created a hostile school environment that could evoke oppositional behavior in students, such as trying to "beat" the tests. On March 13, 2008, the state supreme court ruled in favor of the plaintiffs. Speaking for the majority, Justice Robert Sanders stated that random drug testing of students violated their right to privacy and violated the Washington state constitution as well. Sanders added that even though the U.S. Supreme Court had previously ruled in favor of such testing, states are free to interpret their own state constitutions.

> " The University of Georgia has one of the country's strictest drug-testing policies. One positive test results in an athlete being suspended from competition and requires the completion of 20 hours of community service. "

Marked Discrepancies Among Colleges

Even though the NCAA has policies in place for colleges and universities throughout the United States, the organization does not dictate drug policies for individual schools. Instead, it provides a page of suggested guidelines in its annual drug-testing manual and leaves policy-making decisions up to its members. For this reason, policies often vary widely from school to school. For instance, the University of Georgia has one of the country's strictest drug-testing policies. One positive test results in an athlete being suspended from competition and requires the completion of 20 hours of community service. The athlete must then pass 2 more drug tests before being allowed to compete again, and a third failed test results in permanent banishment from the sport. Georgia Institute of Technology (Georgia Tech) also has a drug policy in place, but it is much more lenient. The first time athletes at Georgia Tech test positive for banned drugs, they are sent to counseling. Only after 3 failed tests does an athlete receive a 1-year suspension, but he or she may still have a chance to return and compete with the team.

Yet even Georgia Tech's policy is much stricter than other colleges, many of which either have no drug-testing policies or very weak ones. This was revealed in an investigation by the *Salt Lake Tribune*, which published its findings in February 2009. The investigation found "vast inconsistencies, curious practices and uncertain accountability in the way the nation's major schools at the top-tier Division I-A level administer their programs." One finding was that some athletes who had tested positive went unpunished, such as a student from the University of Idaho. As the *Tribune* article states: "He was not publicly identified or ruled ineligible. He was not banned from competition. He was not even suspended. Instead, he faced only continued periodic testing over the next year, according to school records, and was required to

> **In August 2007 former University of Hawaii football player Ian Sample claimed that school officials and athletes manipulated NCAA-mandated drug tests.**

enroll in a university counseling program. The school 'encouraged' him to notify his parents. Outrageous? Try, unsurprising."[31]

The authors add that some of America's largest and most prominent colleges do not have their own drug-testing programs and instead rely on the random tests administered by the NCAA, which only about 4 percent of athletes ever take. "It's possible—perhaps even likely—that most college athletes will go their entire careers without being tested for steroids and other performance-enhancing drugs," they write. "And in an era when any athletic accomplishment can be called into dispute because of the growing taint of such drugs, questions remain about whether doping in college sports is a problem that remains mostly undetected and unpunished."[32]

Another state whose college athlete drug-testing program has been criticized is Hawaii. In August 2007 former University of Hawaii football player Ian Sample claimed that school officials and athletes manipulated NCAA-mandated drug tests. In a book about the 2006 football season, Sample stated that marijuana was the drug of choice for players, but he was also convinced that some of them took steroids. He wrote: "Have people on the team taken steroids? Yes, they have. Sometimes it's obvious, you see someone improve over a couple months by leaps and bounds—we all know it's naturally impossible. I think it's known but not really talked about." Sample also claimed in the book that random testing was not happening "randomly" at all because the team management selected the athletes who they wanted to test: "The higher ups definitely know what they are doing when they decide who will be tested."[33]

> If tests that detected performance-enhancing drugs had been performed at [Don Hooton's] son's Dallas-area high school during 2003, the young athlete might be alive today.

The Taylor Hooton Tragedy

Of all those who feel strongly about toughening drug-testing policies in America's schools, no one is more passionate than Don Hooton. If tests that detected performance-enhancing drugs had been performed at his son's Dallas-area high school during 2003, the young athlete might be alive today. Taylor Hooton had been a star pitcher on the school's baseball team. When he was 16, his coach recommended that he start taking steroids so he could build muscle and be more competitive during his senior year. Hooton took the coach's advice and began to bulk up quickly—but there were frightening differences as well.

Known as a young man who was friendly, smiled often, was popular in school, and had many, many friends, Hooton's personality changed radically. He often flew into angry rages, during which he pounded the floor with his fists or punched walls, and afterward became tearfully apologetic. He also withdrew several hundred dollars from his parents' bank account without permission. The Hootons became alarmed at their son's uncharacteristic behavior and took him to a doctor for a physical and for drug testing. Hooton was given a clean bill of health, but his parents were not aware of his steroid use, nor did they know that he was only tested for recreational drugs and not steroids. Hooton's behavior continued to worsen, and after he threatened to kill himself, his parents sent him to a psychiatrist. During one of his sessions with the doctor, Hooton confessed that he had been injecting steroids.

Hooton agreed to stop taking the drugs, but his violent mood swings continued. After he stole a digital camera and laptop computer, his family confronted him and said that his behavior was unacceptable. He was grounded and told to stay in his room. The next morning, July 15, 2003, Hooton was found dead in his bedroom, hanging from a noose that he had made out of belts. His death was ruled a suicide, and the Hootons, along with a doctor familiar with the case, are convinced that Taylor's death was related to severe depression that he felt upon discontinuing the use of steroids. "We were caught completely off guard when we lost Taylor," says Don Hooton. "We had no idea the high usage of steroids among our youth. We had no idea of the serious dangers of the drug and we had no experience with suicide itself."[34] To help educate parents and students about the dangers of performance-enhancing drugs, Don Hooton founded the Taylor Hooton Foundation for Fighting Steroid Abuse in honor of his son. One of his hopes is that schools throughout the United States will implement drug-testing policies that are as tough and consistent as those of the Olympics.

No Easy Answers

Opinions about drug testing in high schools and colleges vary widely. On one side of the argument, people like Don Hooton say that such policies are crucial and should be every bit as tough as those of the Olympics. Because of his tragic personal experience, he is also convinced that tough drug policies could save young lives. On the other side are those who insist that drug testing is a violation of individual privacy and is not appropriate for student athletes. So who is right and who is wrong? Since this is an issue that largely revolves around personal opinions, that question may never be answered.

Is More Rigorous Drug Testing Needed for Student Athletes?

It's my opinion that the testing program [in Texas] seems to be working and is a great deterrent to anyone that might be considering using steroids.

—Jeff Fisher, "Texas Lawmakers Re-Examine Steroid Testing Program for High School Athletes," High School Football Huddle, May 4, 2009. http://highschoolfootballhuddle.blogspot.com.

Fisher is a former sports anchor from Fox Sports Net Chicago and WFMZ-TV in Allentown, Pennsylvania, and the creator of a high school football television program called *The Big Ticket*.

I still think it's absolutely ridiculous when states decide to enact high school steroid testing. The vast majority of high schoolers are never going to touch steroids during their athletic career and the ones who do juice are so few that it makes testing seem worthless.

—George Spellwin, "Anabolic Steroid Testing—Texas Spends $6 million and Catches 4 High School Students," Elite Fitness, February 23, 2009. http://bodybuilding.elitefitness.com.

Spellwin is the research director for Elite Fitness, a Web site devoted to bodybuilding.

Bracketed quotes indicate conflicting positions.

* Editor's Note: While the definition of a primary source can be narrowly or broadly defined, for the purposes of Compact Research, a primary source consists of: 1) results of original research presented by an organization or researcher; 2) eyewitness accounts of events, personal experience, or work experience; 3) first-person editorials offering pundits' opinions; 4) government officials presenting political plans and/or policies; 5) representatives of organizations presenting testimony or policy.

" If a steroid test is administered and that parent or student does not want to subject him or herself to it, then they need to realize the gravity of their decision and the consequences that will ensue. There is no gray area here and there shouldn't be. "

—Gregory Moore, "Steroid Test at High School Level a Much Needed Tool," *American Chronicle*, May 29, 2007. www.americanchronicle.com.

Moore is the managing editor of the *San Antonio Informer*, a weekly newspaper that serves the African American community, located in San Antonio, Texas.

" Our goals are to raise awareness among high school and college students and provide more young people with the tools to take a stand against random student drug testing. "

—Drug Policy Alliance Network, "Students Mobilize Against Random Drug Testing," September 9, 2008. www.drugpolicy.org.

The Drug Policy Alliance Network is an organization committed to ending the war on drugs.

" Florida is on the verge of testing high school athletes for steroids. If society really wants to end steroid use, this is the best way to limit it. "

—Peter Golenbock, "Sports Fans on Steroids," *St. Petersburg Times*, June 3, 2007. www.sptimes.com.

Golenbock is an author from St. Petersburg, Florida, who has written a number of sports-related books.

" I never would try to minimize the dangers of steroids. . . . But I've never believed that steroid use is so prevalent in our high schools that we need a statewide testing program. Talk about overkill. "

—David Flores, "Legislature Should Abolish Steroid Tests for High School Athletes," KENS6 San Antonio, May 7, 2009. www.beloblog.com.

Flores is a sports reporter who focuses mainly on high school athletics.

❝School drug testing is not universally supported. . . . Some critics have suggested that the fear of testing may induce adolescents to avoid participating in athletics and other extracurricular activities. . . . Concerns also have been raised that drug testing may lead to other unintended adverse consequences, such as the use of substances that are undetectable by the testing methods used or the employment of strategies to thwart testing.❞

—Chris Ringwalt et al., "Responses to Positive Results from Suspicionless Random Drug Tests in US Public School Districts," *Journal of School Health*, April 2009.

Ringwalt is a researcher at the Chapel Hill Center of the Pacific Institute for Research and Evaluation in North Carolina; the other authors of the study work at institutes in North Carolina and California.

❝I think it's unfortunate the use of steroids has moved down to the high school level. The NCAA started testing for steroids 22 years ago. . . . It's probably time high schools did, too.❞

—Frank Uryasz, interviewed by Joe Smith, "Sports: A Bit of an Inside View on Steroids Testing," *St. Petersburg Times*, July 24, 2007. www.sptimes.com.

Uryasz is the founder of the National Center for Drug Free Sport, which administers drug-testing programs for the NCAA, Minor League Baseball, the NBA, and some high schools.

❝While I believe in protecting the health of all students, including athletes, state-mandated steroid testing is not the way to go.❞

—Ty Meighan, "Mandated Steroid Testing Wrong," *San Angelo (TX) Standard-Times*, March 13, 2007. www.gosanangelo.com.

Meighan is the editorial page editor of the *Standard-Times*.

Facts and Illustrations

Is More Rigorous Drug Testing Needed for Student Athletes?

- In a March 2008 poll conducted by Sacred Heart University, **68 percent** of respondents said that college athletes should be tested for performance-enhancing drugs, and nearly **60 percent** said high school athletes should be tested.

- Only New Jersey, Texas, and Illinois have statewide policies for **drug testing in high schools**.

- Florida ended its high school drug-testing program in 2009 due to the **high expense** and the **low number of positive tests**.

- More than **3,000 drugs** are banned by the National Collegiate Athletic Association, most of which are the same drugs banned in the Olympics.

- The University Interscholastic League, the governing body of high school sports in Texas, has America's largest and most comprehensive drug program, with plans to test between **40,000 and 50,000 student athletes** in all sports between February and the end of each academic year.

- Since Texas implemented its student drug-testing program, only about **3 percent** of the state's 750,000 high school athletes have been tested.

College Athletes Favor Street Drugs over Performance Enhancers

In November 2007 the *Salt Lake Tribune* released the results of an investigative study of drug-testing policies in American colleges and universities. A total of 79 schools furnished information on their programs, and 67 percent of the schools had athletes who tested positive for banned substances. Another finding, however, was that far fewer college athletes use performance enhancers than other types of drugs.

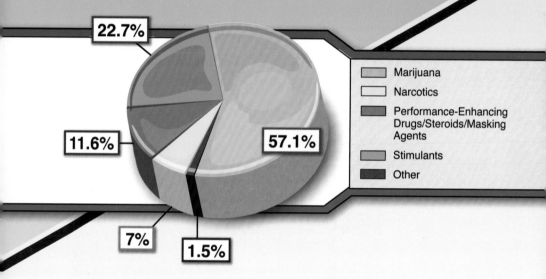

22.7%

11.6%

57.1%

7%

1.5%

Marijuana

Narcotics

Performance-Enhancing Drugs/Steroids/Masking Agents

Stimulants

Other

Total is slightly less than 100 percent due to rounding

Source: *Salt Lake Tribune*, "Collegiate Drug Testing: A National Survey," November 18, 2007. http://extras.sltrib.com.

- Some anabolic steroids are detectable through testing up to **nine months after their use**.

- Texas's drug-testing program costs the state approximately **$6 million** per year.

- An April 2008 report published in the *American Journal of Public Health* showed that almost all school districts randomly test athletes, and **65 percent** randomly test other students engaged in extracurricular activities.

High Support for Student Drug Testing

Although many people object to random drug testing of high school and college athletes, a March 2008 poll by Sacred Heart University in Connecticut showed strong support for such tests. In fact, the percentage of participants who think drug testing should be done at the college level was slightly higher than for the professional level.

Testing for performance-enhancing drugs in sports should occur for athletes in . . .

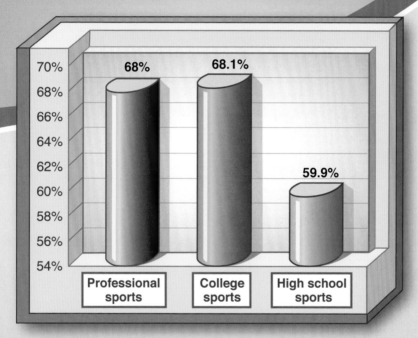

Source: Sacred Heart University, "Americans Say One-Third of Professional Athletes on Performance Enhancing Drugs," March 2008. www.sacredheart.edu.

- The federal government allocates nearly **$12 million** annually for grants to help schools implement drug-testing programs.

- There are currently about **4,200 drug-testing programs** in place at schools throughout the United States.

Student Drug Testing Is Expensive

As of August 2009, only 3 U.S. states mandated drug testing of high school athletes. Cost is one reason so few states test for drugs. In Texas, for instance, a single positive test cost $157,894. And in Florida, where the testing program was deemed too expensive, the testing program was dropped in February 2009. The table shows program costs and results for 4 states, including Florida before it canceled its program.

State	Number of student drug tests performed	Number of athletes who tested positive	Cost
Texas	45,193 from February 2008 through May 2009	19	$6 million
New Jersey	1,500 over a three-year period	2	$300,000
Illinois	684 during the 2008-2009 school year	0	$150,000
Florida	600 during the 2007-2008 school year	1	$100,000

Source: Brian Alexander, "Student Steroid Tests Get an 'F,' Say Some Experts," MSNBC, August 26, 2009. www.msnbc.msn.com.

- An investigative report by the *Salt Lake Tribune* showed that only about **4 percent** of college athletes are tested under the NCAA's drug-testing program.

Number of Student Drug-Testing Programs Growing

According to a January 2009 report by the White House Office of National Drug Control Policy, the popularity of student drug-testing programs is "exploding" across the United States. Even though only Texas, New Jersey, and Illinois, have statewide mandatory drug-testing legislation in place, school districts throughout the country have been implementing their own policies.

States with school districts that have student drug-testing programs in place, 2008

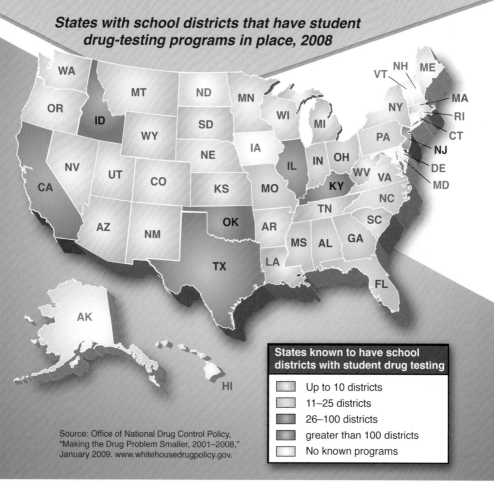

States known to have school districts with student drug testing

- Up to 10 districts
- 11–25 districts
- 26–100 districts
- greater than 100 districts
- No known programs

Source: Office of National Drug Control Policy, "Making the Drug Problem Smaller, 2001–2008," January 2009. www.whitehousedrugpolicy.gov.

Should Drug Use Be Legalized in Competitive Sports?

66In the same way that we have learned about injury prevention and safety equipment, we need performance drugs exposed to the hot light of public scrutiny. We need to legitimize their use.99

—Kate Schmidt, a former U.S. Olympic javelin thrower.

66I am not willing to pay the price for legalizing steroids and performance-enhancing drugs, because I've seen too often what it can do. I don't want to go to the cemetery and tell all the athletes who are dead there, hey guys, soon you'll have a lot more of your friends coming, because we're going to legalize this stuff.99

—George Michael, the creator and former host of *Sports Machine* on NBC News.

Whether referring to illicit drugs such as marijuana or performance-enhancing drugs such as steroids, the issue of legalization is rife with controversy. Many are adamantly opposed to legalization, arguing that if drugs were legal they would be easier for people to get, which could cause steroid use to soar especially among student athletes. They also argue that athletic performance should be the result of training and hard work and that performance-enhancing drugs give users an unfair advantage over others who choose not to take drugs.

This, they insist, is cheating and should not be allowed in any sport.

Yet people who want performance-enhancing drugs legalized have their own reasons for believing the way they do. Many insist that adult athletes should be able to decide for themselves whether to take the drugs and that using them is nothing more than another way to build up the body and be more competitive. Many athletes take multivitamins, eat high-protein diets, and take nutritional supplements—all of which are aimed at enhancing power, speed, and endurance. So, legalization proponents ask, why should performance-enhancing drugs be singled out as wrong? As an article on CBS Sports.com about the use of steroids among baseball players states:

> Major League Baseball should legalize steroids and end this madness once and for all. . . . If anything, legalizing steroids will give the sports world a more clear view of athletes and the values they stand for. Getting this issue out in the open where it can be discussed as well as researched thoroughly would clear up misconceptions as well as provide a potentially safer way for people who decide to partake in this activity.[35]

Congress Makes Steroids Illegal

During the mid-1980s it was brought to the attention of Congress that anabolic steroid use was rampant in professional and amateur sports. Use of the drugs was also alleged to be reaching epidemic proportions among student athletes. Congressional hearings were held between 1988 and 1990 in order to determine the seriousness of the problem and examine whether steroids should be included in the Controlled Substances Act along with illicit drugs such as heroin and cocaine. Witnesses who testified at the hearings included representatives from the Food and Drug Administration, the Drug Enforcement Administration, and the National Institute on Drug Abuse, as well as a number of medical professionals. According to New York attorney Rick Collins, many of these witnesses recommended that the legislation not be amended to include steroids. He writes: "Even the American Medical Association repeatedly and vehemently opposed it, maintaining that abuse of these hormones does not lead to the physical or psychological dependence required for scheduling under the Controlled Substances Act."[36]

Collins adds that records from the hearings suggest that Congress was not so concerned about the addictive or potentially harmful properties of steroids. Rather, the main concern expressed about the drugs was that athletes who take them have an unfair advantage over athletes who do not. Many witnesses who were called to testify at the hearings were representatives from competitive athletics. Their perspective was that steroids should be banned because athletes who take them are cheating, and making this legal was unfair to "clean" athletes who stay away from drugs. Congress agreed, and the Anabolic Steroid Control Act of 1990 made anabolic steroids a Schedule III controlled substance effective as of February 27, 1991. Since that time steroids have only been legal if they are prescribed by a doctor for treating medical conditions. "Those caught illegally possessing anabolic steroids even for purely personal use," writes Collins, "face arrest and prosecution. Under the Control Act, it is unlawful for any person knowingly or intentionally to possess an anabolic steroid unless it was obtained directly, or pursuant to a valid prescription or order, from a practitioner, while acting in the course of his professional practice."[37]

> "Many are adamantly opposed to legalization, arguing that if drugs were legal they would be easier for people to get, which could cause steroid use to soar.

The Case for Legalization

Collins is one individual who strongly believes that steroids should be legalized. He maintains that even though the health risks were not Congress's main reason for making the drugs illegal, the danger of steroids *is* the primary argument used to argue against legalization. He says that the potential risk of steroids has been vastly overblown, and studies have shown that the drugs are nowhere near as harmful as is often claimed. "Despite a virtually one-sided presentation in the lay press," writes Collins, "the position that anabolic steroids are such dangerous substances as to warrant militaristic government enforcement tactics is surprisingly controversial. Mounting research strongly suggests that the actual health risks have been overstated to the public."[38]

Collins refers to drugs that are commercially available, such as alcohol and nicotine, as well as over-the-counter drugs such as ibuprofen and aspirin. Together these legal substances are responsible for thousands of deaths each year, and tens of thousands of hospitalizations. Yet steroids are illegal and those drugs are not, which Collins says makes no sense. He also gives examples of other lifestyle choices that are even more potentially harmful than steroids, but they are not forbidden under the law. "Although the inherent risks of dangerous sports and cosmetic surgery are unnecessary," Collins adds, "and may well outweigh the benefits, we do not proscribe these activities. Is it appropriate, then, to prevent mature, informed adults from choosing cosmetic enhancement through physician-administered hormones?"[39]

Former Olympian Kate Schmidt agrees that steroids should be legalized, and she also believes that Olympic athletes should be allowed to use them. As the Marion Jones situation illustrates, athletes who violate Olympic drug bans are strictly punished and sometimes are stripped of any medals they have won. Soon after Jones confessed to taking steroids, Schmidt published an article in the *Dallas Morning News* expressing her viewpoints. She was angry about how Jones was treated, writing: "It sickened me this month to listen to star track-and-fielder Marion Jones admit her steroid use—and have to apologize to everyone she loved for lying to them and letting them down. She was arguably the greatest female sprinter in our history, and thanks at least in part to our own hypocrisy, her reputation has been destroyed."[40]

> The Anabolic Steroid Control Act of 1990 made anabolic steroids a Schedule III controlled substance effective as of February 27, 1991.

Schmidt feels strongly that the public's criticism of Jones and other athletes who use performance-enhancing drugs is unfair. In her article she stated that expectations for athletes are so high that it is not surprising that they would turn to steroids in an effort to become stronger, faster, and better—and that this will most certainly continue. "The genie is out of the bottle," she wrote, "for good." Schmidt's contention is that instead of keeping steroids a banned substance, legalizing them would be a smarter choice. "By accepting these currently banned substances as mainstream," she wrote, "doctors, parents, athletes and coaches could acquire a greater knowledge and understanding of them. Use could be made much safer, clinical trials could be performed and dangerous overuse curbed."[41]

> **Former Olympian Kate Schmidt agrees that steroids should be legalized, and she also believes that Olympic athletes should be allowed to use them.**

Schmidt's reference to making drugs safer is a key point in the argument on behalf of legalizing performance-enhancing drugs. If they were legalized, advocates say, this would put an end to illegal drug trafficking of steroids, which is often how athletes obtain them. The drugs would also be under the control of the U.S. Food and Drug Administration, which would ensure that they are safe. According to ethics professors Bennett Foddy and Julian Savulescu, because steroids are illegal, the focus is on making them undetectable in tests, rather than safe. They write:

> Performance enhancers are produced or bought on the black market and administered in a clandestine, uncontrolled way with no monitoring of the athlete's health. Allowing the use of performance enhancers would make sport safer as there would be less pressure on athletes to take unsafe enhancers and a pressure to develop new safe performance enhancers and to make existing enhancers more effective at safe dosages.[42]

The Case Against Legalization

Most people who believe performance-enhancing drugs should be legalized are passionate about their beliefs—and equally passionate are those who strongly disagree with them. Opponents' arguments range from the perspective that an athlete whose body is pumped up by steroids is a cheater, to the fear that more and more athletes could suffer harmful side effects from taking the drugs. If steroids were legal, increasing numbers of people would be able to obtain them for reasons that are not medical. Thomas Murray, director of the bioethics research institute the Hastings Center, has a number of reasons for objecting to the legalization of steroids. One is that if the drugs became legal, the beauty of athletics would be forever tarnished. As he writes: "We may lose whatever is most graceful, beautiful, and admirable about sport."[43]

Murray adds that performance-enhancing drugs should remain banned in sports for several other reasons:

> respect for the rules of sports, recognition that natural talents and their perfection are the point of sports, and the prospect of an "arms race" in athletic performance. . . . Sports that revere records and historical comparisons (think of baseball and home runs) would become unmoored by drug-aided athletes obliterating old standards. Athletes, caught in the sport arms race, would be pressed to take more and more drugs, in ever wilder combinations and at increasingly higher doses.

If that happened, Murray warns that this could potentially lead to "a slow-motion public health catastrophe."[44]

Many who want performance-enhancing drugs to remain illegal feel that way because they worry about young athletes. If the drugs were legalized, opponents say, they would be much more accessible to teenagers than they are today. This could lead to widespread drug use and increased addictions among young people. Steven Dowshen, a pediatrician from Wilmington, Delaware, explains: "A lot of people tell themselves they'll only use steroids for a season or a school year.

> " **Most people who believe performance-enhancing drugs should be legalized are passionate about their beliefs—and equally passionate are those who strongly disagree with them.** "

Unfortunately, steroids can be addictive, making it hard to stop taking them."[45]

Many medical professionals and antidrug organizations warn against the potential health risks of steroids for anyone who uses them. But the risk is even greater to young people who use the drugs. Even Collins, who is in favor of legalizing the drugs, acknowledges the risk to youth. He writes: "Anabolic steroids can have adverse effects upon the body, with particular risks for teenagers, who are more likely than adults to abuse anabolic steroids in dangerously high dosages and without any medical supervision."[46] According to the National Institute on Drug Abuse, testosterone and other sex hormones rise during puberty, which triggers a growth spurt and also provides the signals to stop bone growth naturally. But when a child or adolescent takes anabolic steroids, sex hormone levels become artificially high. This can prematurely signal the bones to stop growing and result in stunted growth.

> **Legalization opponents fear that if increasing numbers of youth take steroids, the suicide rate could climb even higher.**

Another risk when young people take steroids is severe mood swings and depression. The teenage years generally entail bouts of uncertainty and moodiness. It is also a time when young people become obsessed with body image. Those who are against legalizing performance-enhancing drugs say that because teenagers would be able to obtain them more easily if they were legal, this would inevitably result in wider steroid use among young people. Thus, natural teenage moodiness could be enhanced and lead to feelings of despair and hopelessness. This is of special concern because teenagers are already at relatively high risk of suicide. According to U.S. government studies, suicide is the third leading cause of death among those who are 15 to 24 years old. Legalization opponents fear that if increasing numbers of youth take steroids, the suicide rate could climb even higher.

The Battle Rages On

People have been arguing about drug legalization for decades, and the debate over performance-enhancing drugs is no exception. Some believe that if the drugs were legalized, this would stop illegal steroid trafficking and ensure that the drugs are safer for those who use them. Many also argue that steroids should be legal because Olympic and professional athletes have the right to decide for themselves whether to take them. At the opposite end of the spectrum are those who say performance-enhancing drugs need to remain illegal because they result in athletes cheating, which is unfair to athletes who do not use drugs. Opponents also point out that the drugs pose dangerous risks to athletes' health. It is likely that this debate will continue into the future. Advocates will keep fighting for performance-enhancing drugs to be legalized, and opponents will fight to keep that from happening.

Should Drug Use Be Legalized in Competitive Sports?

> **There's nothing wrong with a knowledgeable adult using steroids to enhance his physique and build muscle mass. In fact, I think it's incredibly stupid that lawmakers haven't legalized steroids in many nations since there are far more dangerous and widely available substances.**

—George Spellwin, "Anabolic Steroid Testing—Texas Spends $6 million and Catches 4 High School Students," Elite Fitness, February 23, 2009. http://bodybuilding.elitefitness.com.

Spellwin is the research director for Elite Fitness, a Web site devoted to body-building.

> **Among some there is an attitude of resignation and self-justification that drugs are just part of sport. They're not. They are part of cheating, part of dirty sport, part of everything that the Olympic spirit is not.**

—Craig Lord, "You Wearing the Right (Wrong) Suit and Genes?" *Swimmers World*, May 2, 2008. http://sportsanddrugs.procon.org.

Lord is the swimming correspondent for the British publication the *Sunday Times*.

* Editor's Note: While the definition of a primary source can be narrowly or broadly defined, for the purposes of Compact Research, a primary source consists of: 1) results of original research presented by an organization or researcher; 2) eyewitness accounts of events, personal experience, or work experience; 3) first-person editorials offering pundits' opinions; 4) government officials presenting political plans and/or policies; 5) representatives of organizations presenting testimony or policy.

66 **I don't think Congress should forcibly allow performance enhancing substances in sports any more than I think Congress should prohibit them.** 99

> —Radley Balko, "Should We Allow Performance Enhancing Drugs in Sports?" *Reason*, January 23, 2008.
> www.reason.com.

Balko is the senior editor for the libertarian publication *Reason* magazine.

66 **The removal of doping controls would have major benefits: less cheating, increased solidarity and respect between athletes, more focus on sport and not on rules.** 99

> —Bennett Foddy and Julian Savulescu, "Ethics of Performance Enhancement in Sport: Drugs and Gene Doping,"
> *Principles of Health Care Ethics*, June 2007. http://sportsanddrugs.procon.org.

Foddy is a bioethics professor at Princeton University, and Savulescu is a professor of practical ethics at the University of Oxford.

66 **If doping is legalized . . . [cycling's] richest riders and teams will have access to techniques that lesser lights don't. The playing field, never level, would be tilted permanently.** 99

> —Joe Lindsey, "Con to the Question '*Should Performance Enhancing Drugs (Such as Steroids) Be Accepted in Sports?*'
> ProCon.org, October 23, 2008. http://sportsanddrugs.procon.org.

Lindsey is a contributing writer for *Bicycling* magazine.

66 **Fans come to see Herculean efforts and the fact that competitors may have used drugs has not deterred record attendances. The fans want to be entertained and the popularly held belief that all athletes take drugs has not deterred attendees.** 99

> —Anthony P. Millar, "Should Drug Testing Be Banned?" *Doping Journal*, April 19, 2007.
> http://sportsanddrugs.procon.org.

Millar is the director of research at the Lewisham Sports Medicine Institute in the United Kingdom.

66 We have not come close to determining the extent of performance-enhancing drugs in baseball. Yet, despite the disclosures and innuendo, fans are flocking to baseball games in record numbers. Where's the outrage? There is none. 99

—William C. Rhoden, "Sports of the Times; Fans Tolerate Doing, and Media Remain Riveted," *New York Times*, May 26, 2007. http://query.nytimes.com.

Rhoden is a sports columnist for the *New York Times*.

66 In cycling, doping allegations can instantly tarnish a sponsor's reputation—and make it difficult to draw new multinational companies into the sport. 99

—Raf Casert, "Continued Doping Scandals Have Some Cycling Sponsors Backpedaling," *USA Today*, December 14, 2007. http://sportsanddrugs.procon.org.

Casert is a sports writer for the Associated Press.

Facts and Illustrations

Should Drug Use Be Legalized in Competitive Sports?

- A College of New Jersey survey of teenagers that was published in March 2008 showed that **60 percent** of steroid users and **29 percent** of nonusers thought that using steroids for athletic purposes was legal.

- In a March 2008 poll conducted by Sacred Heart University, **69 percent** of respondents said that Congress was wasting time and taxpayer dollars investigating performance-enhancing drugs in baseball and other sports.

- In a September 2007 poll by the Institute for Ethics and Emerging Technologies, **53 percent** of respondents said that steroids should be banned in professional sports.

- In October 2008 Congress unanimously passed a bill that increases the maximum sentence for illegally selling anabolic steroids from **5 years to 10 years**, and up to **15 years if the drug causes death or serious injury**.

- A poll posted in August 2009 by Elite Fitness showed that **32 percent** of respondents thought all steroids should remain illegal, and **29 percent** thought only certain types of steroids should be legalized.

- A 2009 survey by Condition Nutrition showed that **80 percent** of extreme sports athletes (mostly mixed martial arts) were addicted to steroids.

Americans Want Steroids Banned in Professional Sports

The issue of legalizing performance-enhancing drugs is fraught with controversy. Some say the drugs should be legalized while others adamantly disagree. During a September 2007 poll by the Institute for Ethics & Emerging Technologies, participants shared their thoughts about steroids in professional sports, with most favoring a ban.

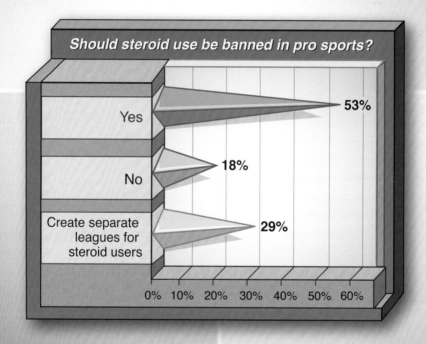

Should steroid use be banned in pro sports?

Source: Institute for Ethics & Emerging Technologies, "Poll: Should Steroids Be Banned in Pro-Sports?" September 30, 2007. http://ieet.org.

- As of December 2008 the World Anti-Doping Agency had banned **192 performance-enhancing drugs** for Olympic athletes, including steroids and HGH.

- During a February 2009 poll by the Student Educational Exchange, participants were asked if it is important for steroids to remain illegal in major league sports; **79 percent** answered yes, **14 percent** said no, and **6 percent** were not sure.

PED Enforcement Costs Time and Money

One of the arguments in support of legalizing performance-enhancing drugs is that legalization would end black market trafficking of the drugs, which the Drug Enforcement Administration says is a serious and costly problem. Enforcing laws against PED use, other than for medical conditions, takes huge amounts of time and money. One such effort, *Operation Raw Deal*, ended in 2007. Described as the largest steroids sting operation in U.S. history, it involved the seizure of 56 laboratories that produced anabolic steroids and human growth hormone in states across the country.

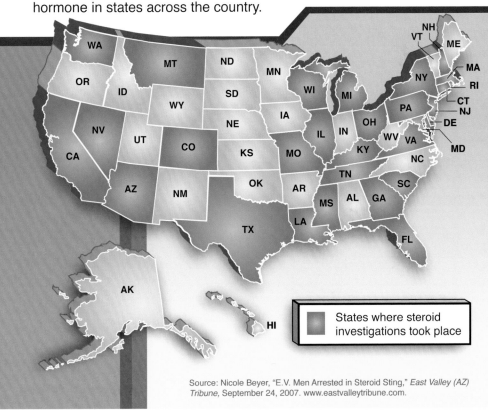

States where steroid investigations took place

Source: Nicole Beyer, "E.V. Men Arrested in Steroid Sting," *East Valley (AZ) Tribune*, September 24, 2007. www.eastvalleytribune.com.

- In a survey posted on the Web site Condition Nutrition in April 2009, nearly **62 percent** of respondents stated that over-the-counter health and nutrition products should not be regulated by the Food and Drug Administration.

Today's Teens Have Less Access to Steroids

Concern about increased access for young athletes is one reason many people oppose the legalization of performance-enhancing drugs. According to a 2008 study by researchers from the University of Michigan's Institute for Social Research, about a third of twelfth graders surveyed say they can easily get steroids. That percentage, however, is significantly less than in 1992, when nearly half of twelfth graders surveyed said it was easy to get steroids.

Changing trend in steroid availability from 1992 to 2008 as perceived by twelfth graders

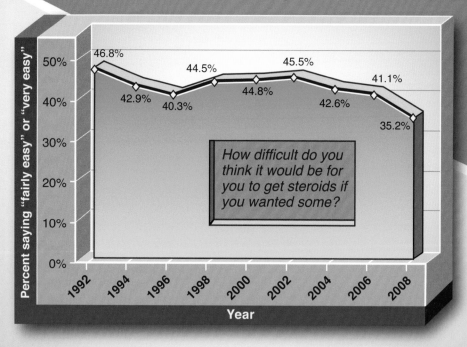

Source: Lloyd D. Johnston et al., *Monitoring the Future: National Results on Adolescent Drug Use*, May 2009. http://monitoringthefuture.org.

- In a survey of more than 3,200 students that was published in March 2008, **57 percent** of steroid users and **12 percent** of nonusers said they believe professional athletes have the right to use steroids.

- A survey posted on the Bleacher Report Web site in February 2009 showed that **64.5 percent** of respondents believe steroids should not be allowed in professional sports, **30.6 percent** believed that they should, and **4.8 percent** were not sure.

- A 2007 study of U.S. weight-loss and athletic supplements by the British laboratory HFL Sport Science found that steroids were contained in **25 percent** of the 52 products analyzed.

Key People and Advocacy Groups

American College of Sports Medicine (ACSM): The largest sports medicine and exercise science organization in the world, the ACSM denounces the use of performance-enhancing drugs by athletes and advocates for more aggressive, random testing.

Bay Area Laboratory Cooperative (BALCO): A sports nutrition company that was founded in 1984 to sell legal food supplements and do chemical testing, BALCO was at the center of a scathing drug scandal. From 2002 to 2004 BALCO was investigated by federal authorities for making and distributing a steroid known as "the Clear," which was not detectable through drug tests. The company's founder, Victor Conte, was indicted in February 2004 and sentenced to 4 months in prison and 4 months of house arrest.

Barry Bonds: A major league outfielder who is currently a free agent, Bonds has been called one of the greatest baseball players in history, and in August 2007 he broke Hank Aaron's record for hitting the most home runs of all time. Bonds's reputation was tarnished, however, because the following November he was indicted on perjury and obstruction of justice charges for allegedly using steroids and lying about it to a grand jury.

International Olympic Committee: An organization that is charged with overseeing the Olympic Games and which states that its number one priority is the fight against the use of prohibited drugs by athletes.

Marion Jones: A five-time Olympic medal–winning sprinter, Jones spent six months in prison for lying to federal investigators about her use of steroids.

George J. Mitchell: A former U.S. senator from Maine who investigated the use of performance-enhancing drugs among Major League Baseball players and developed a comprehensive report to the commissioner of baseball in December 2007.

Dale Murphy: A former Major League Baseball player who founded the antidrug group iWontCheat Foundation.

National Center for Drug Free Sport: An organization that is dedicated to preventing drug use in athletics through drug use prevention services and drug testing.

Richard Pound: A former Olympian and former vice president of the International Olympic Committee who is currently chair of the World Anti-Doping Agency, Pound is one of the most outspoken opponents of the use of performance-enhancing drugs in sports.

Kate Schmidt: A former U.S. Olympic javelin thrower and bronze medal winner who has been outspoken in her belief that performance-enhancing drugs should be legalized.

U.S. Anti-Doping Agency: The national antidrug organization for the Olympic movement in the United States that provides research initiatives and educational programs to help prevent athletes from taking drugs.

Robert Voy: The former chief medical officer and director of sports medicine and science for the U.S. Olympic Committee, Voy is an adamant critic of performance-enhancing drugs being used in sports.

Chronology

1935
A team of German scientists develops anabolic steroids as a treatment for testosterone deficiency, a condition known as hypogonadism.

1990
Congress introduces the Anabolic Steroid Control Act, which raises the crime of steroid trafficking from a misdemeanor to a felony.

1958
The first anabolic steroid in pill form is introduced by Ciba pharmaceuticals. Marketed under the name Dianabol, it is prescribed to promote healing and strength in patients.

1988
After he tests positive for anabolic steroids, Olympic sprinter Ben Johnson is stripped of his gold medal, and his record-setting time is deleted from Olympic record books.

1930

1960

1990

1954
U.S. weight-lifting doctor John Ziegler begins working on a technique to produce a compound with the muscle-building benefits of testosterone and without side effects such as prostate enlargement.

1975
The International Olympic Committee adds anabolic steroids to its list of substances that are banned for athletes.

1969
Sports Illustrated publishes a three-part investigative series entitled "Problems in a Turned-On World," which exposes the widespread use of drugs by elite athletes. Sources cited in the article predict that this drug use will eventually explode into an epidemic.

1963
The San Diego Chargers win the American Football League championship game, and later it is revealed that all the players had been taking anabolic steroids throughout their entire time at training camp.

1986
University of Maryland basketball star Len Bias dies of cardiac arrest after snorting cocaine, prompting some colleges to adopt tougher drug screening programs.

1999
The U.S. Olympic Committee announces the creation of the U.S Anti-Doping Agency, effective October 1, 2000.

2009
Professional baseball slugger Alex Rodriguez admits that he used steroids from 2001 to 2003 when he played with the Texas Rangers.

2003
Marion Jones, a champion sprinter and the winner of five Olympic medals, testifies before federal investigators that she did not take steroids before the 2000 Olympics. Further investigations show that she lied, and she is eventually stripped of her medals and sentenced to six months in prison.

2008
The Professional Golfers' Association implements a drug-testing policy whereby any golfer can be tested at any time or place, during or out of competition, without advance notice.

2000

2010

2001
Congress recognizes the U.S. Anti-Doping Agency as the official antidrug agency for the U.S. Olympics.

2007
Professional wrestler Chris Benoit kills his wife and 7-year-old son and then commits suicide in their home in Fayetteville, Georgia. Investigators learn that a doctor had been providing Benoit with a 10-month supply of anabolic steroids every 3 to 4 weeks, leading many to suspect that this had caused psychosis and what is known as "roid rage."

2004
Victor Conte, founder of the Bay Area Laboratory Cooperative (BALCO), is indicted for making a steroid that is undetectable in blood tests and distributing the drug to elite athletes. He is sentenced to four months in prison and four months of house arrest.

2005
The book *Juiced: Wild Times, Rampant 'Roids, Smash Hits, & How Baseball Got Big* by José Canseco is released. In the book Canseco, a professional baseball player, reveals his own use of steroids starting at age 20, and he claims that up to 85 percent of major league players use performance-enhancing drugs.

Related Organizations

Association Against Steroid Abuse

521 N. Sam Houston Pkwy. East, Suite 635

Houston, TX 77060

phone: (281) 999-9934

Web site: www.steroidabuse.com

The Association Against Steroid Abuse seeks to educate the public and safeguard against the abuse of anabolic steroids. Its Web site features a "Steroids 101" section with a great deal of information, as well as steroid statistics, the dangers of steroid abuse, steroid use in high schools, steroid myths, and true stories of steroid abuse.

Drug Policy Alliance Network

70 W. Thirty-sixth St., 16th Floor

New York, NY 10018

phone: (212) 613-8020 • fax: (212) 613-8021

e-mail: nyc@drugpolicy.org • Web site: www.drugpolicy.org

The Drug Policy Alliance Network is an organization that is committed to ending the war on drugs and is staunchly against random drug testing in high schools and colleges. Its Web site offers a collection of news articles, a searchable library, position papers, and a link to the D'Alliance blog.

International Association of Athletics Federations (IAAF)

17 rue Princesse Florestine, BP 359

MC98007, Monaco

phone: 011-377-93 10 88 • fax: 011-377-93 15 9515

e-mail: info@iaaf.org • Web site: www.iaaf.org

The IAAF strives to ensure that athletics continues to play a leading role throughout the world for the benefit of all athletes, fans, and enthusiasts. Its Web site features news articles, statistics, downloadable newsletters, and a special "Anti-Doping" section.

International Olympic Committee

Château de Vidy

1007 Lausanne

Switzerland

phone: 011-41-21-621-6111 • fax: 011-41-21-621-6216

Web site: www.olympic.org

The International Olympic Committee is charged with overseeing the Olympic Games and states that its number one priority is the fight against the use of prohibited drugs by athletes. Its Web site offers numerous publications, including one entitled *The Fight Against Doping and Promotion of Athletes' Health*, as well as newsletters, news articles, and a list of all Olympic medal winners since 1896.

iWontCheat Foundation

31351 Via Colinas, Suite 204

Westlake Village, CA 91362

phone: (805) 480-1387

e-mail: dale@iwontcheat.com • Web site: http://iwontcheat.com

Founded by former professional baseball player Dale Murphy, the iWontCheat Foundation seeks to provide schools, youth sports leagues, and summer camps with a character education program that is designed to confront what it perceives as the growing epidemic of dishonesty throughout society. Its Web site features an "iWontCheat in the News" section, links to articles, audio clips, and an ABC News video.

National Center for Drug Free Sport

2537 Madison Ave.

Kansas City, MO 64108

phone: (816) 474-8655 • fax: (816) 502-9287

e-mail: info@drugfreesport.com • Web site: www.drugfreesport.com

The National Center for Drug Free Sport is dedicated to preventing drug use in athletics through drug-use prevention services and drug testing. Its Web site offers a wide variety of information, including a banned/ prescription drug database, a "Drugs of Abuse" section, news releases, the quarterly *Insight* newsletter, and a comprehensive "National Headlines" section that links to national news stories about drugs and sports.

National Collegiate Athletic Association (NCAA)

700 W. Washington St.

PO Box 6222

Indianapolis, IN 46206-6222

phone: (317) 917-6222 • fax: (317) 917-6888

Web site: www.ncaa.org

The NCAA is a voluntary organization through which America's colleges and universities govern their athletics programs. Its Web site offers news releases, articles, statistics, a list of banned drugs, information about drug testing, and a list of penalties for student athletes who take banned drugs.

National Institute on Drug Abuse (NIDA)

National Institutes of Health

6001 Executive Blvd., Room 5213

Bethesda, MD 20892-9561

phone: (301) 443-1124

e-mail: information@nida.nih.gov • Web site: www.nida.nih.gov

The NIDA supports research efforts and ensures the rapid dissemination of research in order to improve prevention, treatment, and policy as it relates to drug abuse and addiction. Its Web site has a special section for students and young adults called "NIDA for Teens" that offers a wealth of information about drugs, including performance-enhancing drugs.

U.S. Anti-Doping Agency

1330 Quail Lake Loop, Suite 260

Colorado Springs, CO 80906-4651

phone: (719) 785-2000; toll-free: (866) 601-2632

fax: (719) 785-2001

Web site: www.usantidoping.org

The U.S. Anti-Doping Agency, which is the national anti-doping organization for the Olympic Movement in the United States, provides research initiatives and educational programs to help prevent athletes from taking drugs. Its Web site offers information about the dangers of steroid use, as well as statistics, news releases, frequently asked questions, and the *Spirit of Sport* newsletter.

U.S. Olympic Committee

1 Olympic Plaza

Colorado Springs, CO 80909-5760

phone: (719) 866-4444

e-mail: media@usoc.org • Web site: www.usoc.org

The U.S. Olympic Committee is considered the steward of the U.S. Olympic Movement and acts as the coordinating body for all Olympics-related athletic activity in the country. Its Web site features links to a number of athletes' blogs, news articles, and an "Olympics Facts and Figures" section.

World Anti-Doping Agency (WADA)

Stock Exchange Tower

800 Place Victoria, Suite 1700

Montreal, QC H4Z 1B7, Canada

phone: (514) 904-9232

e-mail: info@wada-ama.org • Web site: www.wada-ama.org

The WADA is an independent international organization that is dedicated to promoting, coordinating, and monitoring the fight against all forms of drug use in sports. Its Web site features news releases, compliance reports, a searchable database of speeches and presentations, research for athletes and anti-doping organizations, and *Play True* magazine.

For Further Research

Books

Shaun Assael, *Steroid Nation: Juiced Home Run Totals, Anti-Aging Miracles, and a Hercules in Every High School: The Secret History of America's True Drug Addiction*. New York: ESPN, 2007.

Laura K. Egendorf, *Performance-Enhancing Drugs*. San Diego: ReferencePoint, 2007.

Mark Fainaru-Wada and Lance Williams, *Game of Shadows: Barry Bonds, BALCO, and the Steroids Scandal That Rocked Professional Sports*. New York: Gotham, 2007.

Jeri Freedman, *Professional Wrestling: Steroids in and out of the Ring*. New York: Rosen Central, 2009.

Jason Porterfield, *Doping: Athletes and Drugs*. New York: Rosen, 2009.

Jennifer L. Skancke and Lauri S. Friedman, *Athletes and Drug Use*. Detroit: Greenhaven/Gale Cengage Learning, 2009.

Annie Leah Sommers, *College Athletics: Steroids and Supplement Abuse*. New York: Rosen, 2010.

Krista West, *Steroids and Other Performance-Enhancing Drugs*. New York: Chelsea House, 2009.

Periodicals

Marky Billson, "Cheating in Baseball Is Old News: The Game Has a Long History of Players and Teams Trying to Gain an Edge, Ranging from Spitballs, Sign-Stealing, Corked Bats, Doctoring Balls, Altering Field Conditions and Using Performance Enhancing Drugs," *Baseball Digest*, May 2008.

Justin Divney, "Steroids in Sports: A Race Between Cheaters and Those Who Wish to Prevent Them," *Earth Focus: One Planet–One Community*, Spring 2007.

Melody K. Hoffman, "Yankees Shortstop Derek Jeter Leads by Example, Steers Kids Away from Drugs," *Jet*, September 17, 2007.

Luis Fernando Llosa and L. Jon Wertheim, "Sins of a Father (Special Report, a Teen on Steroids: In-Line Skater Corey Gahen)," *Sports Illustrated*, January 21, 2008.

Jack McCallum, "The Real Dope: It's Not Just Sports," *Sports Illustrated*, March 17, 2008.

Edwin Moses, "Why Baseball Is in Denial," *Newsweek International*, March 2, 2009.

Joe Posnanski, "Without a Clue (Scorecard: Life on and off the Field," *Sports Illustrated*, June 22, 2009.

Gretchen Reynolds, "Girls & Steroids: These Days More High School Girls Are Abusing Anabolic Steroids. Here's What You Need to Know Now," *Seventee*n, August 2008.

Ron Sirak, "The Truth About Testing: As Pro Golf Joins Other Major Sports in Testing Competitors, Recreational Drugs, Not Steroids, Raise Red Flags for Insiders," *Golf World*, January 11, 2008.

Kirsten Weir, "Big Dopes: Athletes Who Take Performance-Enhancing Drugs Risk Their Reputations and Their Health," *Current Science: A Weekly Reader Publication*, January 4, 2008.

Internet Sources

Radley Balko, "Should We Allow Performance Enhancing Drugs in Sports?" *Reason*, January 23, 2008. www.reason.com/news/show/124 577.html.

Arthur Caplan, "A Shot in the Rear: Why Are We Really Against Steroids?" Science Progress, March 13, 2008. www.scienceprogress.org/2008/03/a-shot-in-the-rear.

Jeffrey Katz, "Should We Accept Steroid Use in Sports?" National Public Radio, January 23, 2008. www.npr.org/templates/story/story.php?storyId=18299098&sc=emaf.

George J. Mitchell, *Report to the Commissioner of Baseball of an Independent Investigation into the Illegal Use of Steroids and Other Performance Enhancing Substances by Players in Major League Baseball*, ESPN, December 13, 2007. http://assets.espn.go.com/media/pdf/071213/mitchell_report.pdf.

Source Notes

Overview

1. Quoted in *The Oprah Winfrey Show*, "Former Olympic Medalist Marion Jones' First Interview After Prison," October 29, 2008. www.oprah.com.
2. Daniel Engber, "The Growth Hormone Myth," *Slate*, March 24, 2007. www.slate.com.
3. Michael F. Schafer and Mary Ann Porucznik, "If You're Not Cheating, You're Not Trying," AAOS *Now*, June 2008. www.aaos.org.
4. Quoted in Brittany Stahl, "Despite MLB Scandal, Steroids Rampant in College Baseball," *NYC Pavement Pieces*, March 26, 2009. http://journalism.nyu.edu.
5. George J. Mitchell, *Report to the Commissioner of Baseball of an Independent Investigation into the Illegal Use of Steroids and Other Performance Enhancing Substances by Players in Major League Baseball*, ESPN, December 13, 2007. http://assets.espn.go.com.
6. Quoted in Dave Caldwell, "Bill Would Further Anti-Drug Efforts," *New York Times*, October 3, 2008. www.nytimes.com.
7. Women's Sports Foundation, "Drugs—Athletes and Drug Use: The Foundation Position," 2008. www.womenssportsfoundation.org.
8. Quoted in Shaun Assael, "High School Testing Loses Momentum," *ESPN*, March 5, 2009. http://sports.espn.go.com.
9. Zev Chafets, "Let Steroids into the Hall of Fame," *New York Times*, June 19, 2009. www.nytimes.com.

How Serious a Problem Is Drug Use Among Athletes?

10. Gary Valk, "Letter from the Publisher," *Sports Illustrated*, June 23, 1969. http://sportsillustrated.cnn.com.
11. Jim Bunning, "Steroid Users Have No Place in Hall of Fame," *U.S. News & World Report*, July 21, 2009. www.usnews.com.
12. Steve Lyons, "Hall of Fame Should Get Over the Steroid Scandal—Cheating Is Common," *U.S. News & World Report*, July 21, 2009. www.usnews.com.
13. Quoted in Michael Sokolove, "Drug Use Brings Doubt to Olympic Performances," August 7, 2008. www.nytimes.com.
14. Wayne Coffey, "Teens' Big Worry: For High School Athletes, Steroids Still the Rage," *New York Daily News*, December 16, 2007. www.nydailynews.com.
15. Quoted in BBC News, "Bodybuilder Scarred from Steroids," August 21, 2008. http://news.bbc.co.uk.
16. Alan D. Rogol, "Testimony: Myths and Facts About Human Growth Hormone, B-12, and Other Substances," Endocrine Society, February 12, 2008. http://oversight.house.gov.
17. Bob Smizik, "Make Punishment Fit the Crime," *Pittsburgh Post-Gazette*, May 8, 2009. http://community.post-gazette.com.

How Effective Are Drug-Testing Policies?

18. Quoted in Eddie Pells, "Mayfield Case Puts Spotlight on NASCAR Drug Policy," ABC News, July 10, 2009. http://abcnews.go.com.
19. Quoted in Pells, "Mayfield Case Puts Spotlight on NASCAR Drug Policy."
20. Quoted in Joseph White, "Congress Raises Possibility of Drug-Testing

Law," *Sporting News*, February 27, 2008. www.sportingnews.com.

21. Edwin Moses, "Why Baseball Is in Denial," *Newsweek International*, March 2, 2009.

22. Lester Munson, "Congressional Hearing Takes Aim at Drug Legislation," ESPN, February 26, 2008. http://sports.espn.go.com.

23. Quoted in Mark Maske, "Other Leagues Back NFL in StarCaps Case," *Washington Post* NFL News Feed, July 22, 2009. http://views.washingtonpost.com.

24. Frank Uryasz, "Guest Editorial: Stay Current on Drug Testing," National Collegiate Athletic Association, June 4, 2007. www.ncaa.org.

25. Quoted in Uryasz, "Guest Editorial."

26. Annie Vernon et al., letter to the World Anti-Doping Agency, The Rowing Service, February 2009. www.rowingservice.com.

27. Vernon et al., letter to the World Anti-Doping Agency.

Is More Rigorous Drug Testing Needed for Student Athletes?

28. Clarence Thomas, *Board of Education of Independent School District No. 92 of Pottawatomie County v. Earls*, Cornell University Law School, June 27, 2002. www4.law.cornell.edu.

29. Quoted in Jason Blevins, "Schools Say Yes to Drug Testing," *Denver Post*, May 26, 2008. www.denverpost.com.

30. Quoted in Blevins, "Schools Say Yes to Drug Testing."

31. Michael C. Lewis and Nate Carlisle, "Broken College System Lets Drug Cheats Slip Through the Cracks," *Salt Lake Tribune*, February 2, 2009. www.sltrib.com.

32. Lewis and Carlisle, "Broken College System Lets Drug Cheats Slip Through the Cracks."

33. Quoted in *USA Today*, "Ex Hawaii WR Alleges NCAA Drug Tests 'Not Random,'" August 21, 2007. www.usatoday.com.

34. Quoted in U.S. Drug Enforcement Administration, "Steroids and Our Use: An Interview with Don Hooton," June 2006. www.usdoj.gov.

Should Drug Use Be Legalized in Competitive Sports?

35. Thoughts of a Gentledawg, "Legalize Steroids," CBS Sports.com, June 30, 2008. http://sircheeks.blogs.cbssports.com.

36. Rick Collins, "The Anabolic Steroid Control Act: The Wrong Prescription," MESO-Rx, 2005. www.mesomorphosis.com.

37. Collins, "The Anabolic Steroid Control Act."

38. Collins, "The Anabolic Steroid Control Act."

39. Collins, "The Anabolic Steroid Control Act."

40. Kate Schmidt, "Time to Legalize Steroids," *Dallas Morning News*, October 28, 2007. www.dallasnews.com.

41. Schmidt, "Time to Legalize Steroids."

42. Quoted in ProCon.org, "Should Performance Enhancing Drugs (Such as Steroids) Be Accepted in Sports?" June 2007. http://sportsanddrugs.procon.org.

43. Quoted in ProCon.org, "Should Performance Enhancing Drugs (Such as Steroids) Be Accepted in Sports?"

44. Quoted in ProCon.org, "Should Performance Enhancing Drugs (Such as Steroids) Be Accepted in Sports?"

45. Steven Dowshen, "Are Steroids Worth the Risk?" Teens Health, April 2009. http://kidshealth.org .

46. Collins, "The Anabolic Steroid Control Act."

List of Illustrations

Index

About the Author

Peggy J. Parks holds a bachelor of science degree from Aquinas College in Grand Rapids, Michigan, where she graduated magna cum laude. She has written more than 80 nonfiction educational books for children and young adults, as well as published a cookbook called *Welcome Home: Recipes, Memories, and Traditions from the Heart*. Parks lives in Muskegon, Michigan, a town that she says inspires her writing because of its location on the shores of Lake Michigan.